es

up *rvival*

eaturing

IcLeod
Curtis
and
dbetter

gaye croft

For my family

Thomas C. Lothian Pty Ltd
132 Albert Road, South Melbourne, 3205
www.lothian.com.au

National Library of Australia
Cataloguing-in-Publication data:

Croft, Gaye.
  Bosom buddies: uplifting stories of breast cancer survival.

  ISBN 0 7344 0330 5.

  1. Croft, Gaye. 2. Curtis, Diane. 3. Leadbetter, Doris.
  4. McLeod, Sandy. 5. Breast – Cancer – Biography. I. Title.

362.19699449

Cover design and illustration by Georgie Wilson
Text illustrations by Michelle Mackintosh
Text design by David Constable
Typeset by Alena Jençik of Grand Graphix
Printed in Australia by Griffin Press

The specific names of the types of breast cancer of the women in this book
have been intentionally omitted to avoid incorrect self-diagnosis.

The surnames of the doctors, surgeons and specialists in this book have
been intentionally omitted (except where a pseudonym has been used, or
approval has been given for the inclusion of the full name to be used) to
comply with section 64 of the *Medical Practice Act* 1994.

Foreword

For most women, the diagnosis of breast cancer releases an array of emotions. Each will respond in a unique and individual way to this life-changing news.

Bosom Buddies highlights the individual responses of four women and their experiences with breast cancer. The journey from pre-diagnosis through confirmation of disease, treatment options and ongoing survival is conveyed with emotional frankness, openness of spirit and with faith, hope and humour.

I welcome this special book as an insight into the way different women can respond to the diagnosis of breast cancer. The honest revelations found in this text will hopefully reassure other women that they too can be open and individual in expressing their concerns, fears and hopes for the future and that a good laugh with like-minded friends can lighten a day.

Gaye, Sandy, Diane and Doris share a strength in each other and a camaraderie of spirit that is evident in many of those who walk this walk together.

The author of *Bosom Buddies* was a personal inspiration to me during the early years of my involvement with breast cancer patients. Her refreshing humour and candid personality continue to help other women in a support-group setting. To all those wonderful women who are my heroes – keep supporting each other; you do it so well.

Kathleen Murphy
Breast Care Nurse
RN, RM, BNsg, BCN, MRCN

Preface

When I was diagnosed with cancer, it didn't just make me look at death and dying, it made me look at life and living. Life was to be grabbed by the love handles and vigorously hoggled!

My grandmother, Sylvie, used to say, 'If a job's worth doing, it's worth doing well.' My mother used to say, 'And if all your friends jumped off a cliff, would you do that too?'

Looking back at the way I dealt with my diagnosis of cancer, the double mastectomy and breast reconstruction, I didn't jump off a cliff with the others. I didn't want to wear the disguises of a 'cancer patient'. I had no intentions of hiding my baldness or building my bosomless chest up with padding to prove that I was still a woman.

As time and treatments went on, I realised cancer wasn't as intimidating as I had thought it would be. But then, I wasn't *allowing* it to be. My sense of humour remained vibrantly alive. I owned a true acceptance of the situation and felt genuine contentment that manifested itself in my attitude and actions. Many people said I was brave. I simply thought I was doing my job well!

In this book you will find my story, along with the stories of three inspirational women – Sandy, Diane and Doris. While each of our journeys with breast cancer have been different, each of us has tried to maintain our sense of humour throughout, viewing the cancer not as a death or an ordeal, but as an experience.

Breast cancer is increasingly being brought to the fore-front of our attention, and old attitudes are being evaluated. I like to think of it as, 'One small step for man: one giant leap for mamm-kind.'

Breast wishes
Gaye Croft

Contents

Biographies

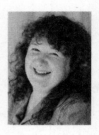

Gaye

Bridal dressmaker. Married to Stephen, with two children: Elissa and Kerrie. Diagnosed in December 1996 at age 32. No family history of breast cancer.

Likes: Getting out of housework.
Dislikes: Housework.

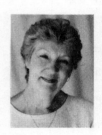

Sandy

Tele-sales rep (now retired). Married to Jim, with four children: Sharon, Mark, Paul and Craig. Diagnosed in 1992 at age 45. Family history of breast cancer in mother.

Sandy's husband had recently become my husband's boss at work. We first met at a 21st party and I loved Sandy immediately. I wanted her to adopt me. About three weeks later she was diagnosed. She is one of my heroes.

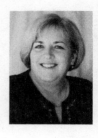

Diane

Ward clerk. Married to Alan, with three children: Craig, Matthew and Phillip. Diagnosed in 1994 at age 39. No family history of breast cancer.

While discussing breast reconstruction with an oncologist, I was put in touch with Diane, as she'd been in a similar position. Diane's story is remarkable. Her incident with a mammogram operator some time after her breast reconstruction still puts me in awe. Diane's attitude is positively amazing.

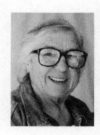

Doris

Professional writer and teacher. Married to Richard, with two children: Vicki and Dominic. Diagnosed in 1965 at age 37; diagnosed in 1988 at age 59. No family history of breast cancer.

During my breast reconstruction, a nurse gave me a poem to read. It was written by Doris Leadbetter – an inspirational woman who wrote humorously about her breast cancer. I thought she would be great for my book, but never dreamed it would be possible to contact her. The day I returned home, a friend called. 'I think I might have someone for your book. She's a friend – and quite a character – her name is Doris Leadbetter.'

One at a Time

When I was thirty-nine
cancer came and went
taking my left breast with it.

I didn't miss it
and I wasn't married
so he didn't miss it.

I took my time finding a false one
(breast, that is, not husband).
I tried a sheepskin breast;
it scattered gravel on a parquet floor.
I thought of buying a birdseed one
but had images of magpies
pursuing me
down the street
with Alfred Hitchcock.
I settled for a plastic breast:
French, sexy, chic.

Two years later I married
and he thought single-breasted wives
as fashionable as his
double-breasted suits.

Twenty-five years on
the other breast went to the same cause.

No longer did I struggle to balance
plastic with person
as the weight we on
(plastic breasts never need to diet).
Now at last I was flat-chested
like Audrey Hepburn
like the Duchess of Windsor
(no woman can be too flat-chested).

Now I wear t-shirts
tank tops
skinny ribs
my husband's shirts

and I don't bounce on my bicycle.

Doris Leadbetter

CHAPTER 1

It's only cancer

(Challenging the negative perception)

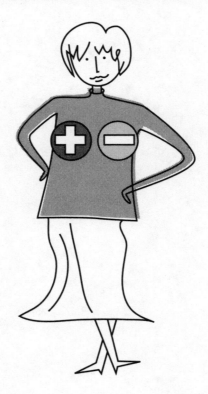

Gaye

Like many, I was fed the fears and horror of cancer from a generation that had watched their loved ones die from the disease with no medical cure.

In those days cancer meant one thing: death.

Since childhood I had always believed that cancer was the worst possible illness you could get. My husband Steve also thought this, having watched his mother die tragically from liver cancer when he was just 17 years old.

Then at the age of 22 Steve was diagnosed with his own cancer – a brain tumour. I was 20 at the time and this was my first close-up, in-your-face experience of cancer. We'd been going out together for four years when Steve had finally asked me to marry him. Two weeks later he was in a hospital bed, surrounded by white coats who were unsure how to remove a cancerous tumour from his brain. Surgery to actually get to the location of the tumour was not an option in this case; it would have caused untold and irreversible damage.

This beautiful young man, who embodied the most natural, easy-going nature, was expected to die.

About a year later, when Steve was recovering, I was astounded when he told me, 'You know Gaye, I don't think it was really *that* bad.'

My opinion of cancer changed dramatically as we went through the experience, and I watched him battle it. I was inspired by the amazing way he handled this life-threatening illness. It made me more aware of the importance of attitude – attitude towards life in general and towards unexpected situations that are thrust upon us. I became aware that even difficult circumstances have their positive moments, and of the possibility of making the most of opportunities within those experiences.

We had our faith, and we saw many wonderful happenings. I prayed a lot. Not out of desperation or as a last resort. Just believing.

After we were married the doctors told us there was 'absolutely no way' that we could have children naturally, and advised Steve, 'Your wife does *not* need to be taking the contraceptive pill.'

But I refused to stop taking it.

I said, 'Crofty, I've prayed about this. If I stop taking the pill we *will* have a baby.'

After Steve's next visit to his team of specialists he came home determined. We went through the whole contraceptive pill discussion again. He put on a puppy face and said, 'Gaye, I don't see the point in you filling your body with chemicals that it doesn't need. It'll give your body a rest. Just for me … *please?*'

So I stopped taking the pill. Because I was halfway through the packet I got my period a couple of days later. Nine months later our first baby was born.

Gaye

My mind boggles when I look back at how all the events unfolded during Steve's illness, and likewise when I got cancer. The choices we made at the time were, in the long run, the right ones for us. And it's only in hindsight that I can see that. You can take so many things for granted, and have no way of knowing the significance of particular situations at the time. Usually it's later (sometimes never) that you realise the extent to which it has helped create the bigger picture.

All this inevitably made it that much easier when it came to handling my own cancer.

I don't dwell on the negativity of why *I* got cancer. At the time I don't even recall thinking, 'Why me?' What intrigued me, after accepting the fact, was a sudden realisation that 'I've got cancer. There is a reason for it. I may never know what the reason is – and yet that doesn't bother me. There is a possibility of dying – well, that's going to happen down the track anyway, cancer or no cancer. The other possibility is living … so in the meantime, I'll do it well!' I do remember thinking that 'whatever develops from this situation is going to be *awesome* … so I'm just going to sit back, relax, and enjoy the ride! The breast may be yet to come!'

Sandy

It's sad that people look at cancer with such a dim view. I mean it's certainly nothing to celebrate, but it is possible to make the most of this really horrendous situation and come out of it a better person at the end of the day.

Obviously everyone has their periods of tears and sadness and they wonder, 'Why has this happened to me?' But once you do come to terms with the idea of cancer you think, 'Okay. I've got it. Let's get on with the treatment, and let's start as quickly as we can – no mucking around.'

It's important to learn what the disease is, so that you can understand it and help others to understand it. I think half the time that's the problem with a lot of family and friends – they're just so frightened by the word 'cancer'.

However, once they see that *you're* coping with it (how comfortable *you* are with the situation) and that you're not afraid to be seen with a bald head or no boobs or whatever, it helps them feel a lot more at ease. They may still be a little reluctant to ask questions though, so I think that's where you as the person with the disease sort of owes it to others to say, 'Look; I'm fine. This is what you see today; tomorrow I could be shit. Today I'm fantastic, I feel great. You take me as you find me.'

And take the good with the bad, because for me nine times out of ten it was a lot more good than it was ever bad.

Diane

Basically, no one would walk in and choose to have cancer, but I have to say it's by no means the worst thing that has ever happened to me. I think that people put a lot of emphasis on the belief that cancer is such a bad diagnosis. There are a lot of other conditions out there that are much worse – seemingly 'simple' conditions such as diabetes. People diagnosed with diabetes have to make *huge* adjustments to their lives. It alters their life *every* day for the rest of their life. Having cancer means that you have to make adjustments of course, but not to the same extent.

I'm acutely aware that it's possible to have a recurrence of breast cancer. I'm also aware that if it returned I'd be in big trouble. It wouldn't be a good thing. However, my quality of life and the way I see life has changed for the better directly because of my experience of cancer. It has given me a greater appreciation of life.

If a breast cancer did recur and my life ended up being shorter than I'm hoping it will be, at least I'd know that the quality of my life has been better than if cancer had passed me by.

Doris

Back when I first got cancer in 1965 nobody talked about it.

My diagnosis was made the day after I showed my doctor the lump in my breast. By the next afternoon the lump was gone, my breast was gone and the cancer was gone. There wasn't even enough time for me to worry! I was back at work in about six weeks and that was it.

The second time it happened, 23 years later, I knew a lot more about it. I was more apprehensive this time, but not terribly so.

I think women are very frightened of the words 'breast cancer' because they're frightened it will happen to them.

Then there are women who have developed this theory about themselves, that 'a woman *is* her breasts,' and that losing your breasts (which always sounds rather careless to me) means the end of your sex life – and the end of you being *you.* Because of these reasons, some women are frightened of having lumps looked at.

I can understand that, because the first time I had a lump I put off seeing the doctor about it for 18 months. But, believe me, if you do feel there is something in there that's not quite right, the best thing to do is see your doctor and get it examined.

Now I say, 'You girls out there … *DO* CHECK YOUR BREASTS!' If you don't want to do it yourself, then get somebody else to do it. Any fellow out there would be *more* than willing to learn how. And remember this: on each breast there is only *one* lump allowed – that's the pinky-brown one in the middle! And if it's *not* right in the middle then that's another problem altogether.' (Probably more serious than breast cancer, I shouldn't wonder.)

CHAPTER 2

Storm in a D cup

(Discovery, Diagnosis and Dealing with it)

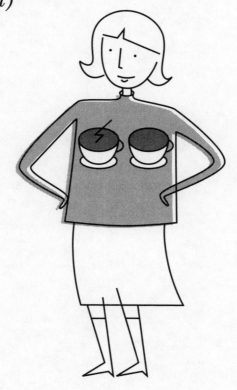

Gaye

By accident, I found the lump in my right breast one night when I was in bed. I quickly searched my other breast to find a matching lump in the same area but I couldn't find anything. Anxiety began to take over and a nauseating coldness prickled through my body. I asked my husband to feel the lump, and sensed his concern at what the most likely outcome might be.

The following morning I made an appointment to see our family doctor and Steve soberly accompanied me.

My GP examined me, and after taking into consideration my mother's medical history of recurrent breast cysts, his prognosis was simply that: it was a cyst. As he finished saying those words I was overcome with a feeling of absolute relief. In synchronsation, Steve flopped back into his chair and released a long, loud, thankful sigh.

Dr Smith explained the alternatives of leaving the cyst or draining it.

'But if it's drained,' I said, 'it will only fill up with fluid again, won't it? Then it'll have to be drained again.'

Smithy agreed. Quickly considering the two

Gaye

options I reassured myself. 'Right. It's not the worst case scenario – CANCER (spelt with capital letters!) Why be masochistic enough to have a needle jabbed in unnecessarily?'

'Don't worry about it then,' I stated nonchalantly.

As we drove home I felt rather pleased with myself. I was 32 years old, I had a cyst in my breast and everything was right with the world.

Five months later I noticed an unusual pain at the location of the cyst. Gently palpating my breast, I realised that the cyst had grown to about two and a half centimetres long and one and a half centimetres wide.

The following day, a Friday, I went to see my doctor again. I wasn't concerned, but this time I'd decided it would be best to drain the fluid so that a biopsy and pathology test could be undertaken.

After examining me, Dr Smith's prognosis echoed my thoughts. 'I'm still convinced it's a cyst,' he assured me, 'but it *has* to be drained.'

He referred me to a specialist, phoning through and booking the appointment himself. They managed to squeeze me in for Monday morning.

'*Terrific!*' I thought sarcastically. 'I've psyched myself up all morning for Smithy to stick this needle into me, and now I have to wait the whole weekend so that a stranger can do it!'

Steve came along with me to see the specialist. We sat in a waiting room and picked over the collection of magazines on the coffee table. Being a dressmaker, I picked up a copy of *Vogue* to read. Les Misérables – Tres Impossible! It was a French edition, printed in 1984. Big hair, big shoulders and lashings of lamé. Great. I picked up an old real-estate brochure and read it through twice, repeating to myself, 'Don't judge the man by his 12-year-old fashion magazines, don't judge the man by his 12-year-old fashion magazines.'

My darling husband is such a vessel of support. He knows how much I dread the thought of having a needle. 'Don't worry, dear,' he said, as he gently patted my leg. 'They're probably running late because the doctor is filing a nice blunt edge on the needle, before he *sticks* it in.'

With that, my beloved kindly relayed all the actions to his commentary – complete with sound effects.

When we were finally ushered into the doctor's office we were welcomed by a comfortable, cheerful atmosphere. The specialist, accompanied by Kathy (a nursing sister specialising in breast problems), made us both feel instantly at ease.

To keep my mind off what was happening while the specialist aspirated (drained) the lump, I told him about a conversation I'd had with my sister, who had just come back to live in Melbourne after spending several years interstate.

One of the first things she had said when she saw me was, 'So, Gaye, when are you going to have a breast reduction?'

With the intention of announcing to my sister that I had indeed had a breast reduction that day, I turned to the specialist as he finished the procedure and asked him how many millilitres of fluid he had drained out of the cyst. (I could use this information as the punch line when I told my sister about my 'reduction'.)

The specialist answered slowly and deliberately. 'Aaahh. It's not a cyst.'

I turned to look at him and focused on the extracted fluid in the vials. It looked more like blood than the murky colour my mother had said was constantly removed from her cysts. The punch line hit me right in the stomach – but I couldn't laugh.

I turned to Steve, knowing that he would offer an expression of confidence. He was staring at the floor, motionless and ashen-faced.

I was to undertake a number of X-rays and ultrasounds the following day to determine what the lump was.

Gaye

As we drove home, I took Steve's hand and said, 'What if it's cancer?'

He wrapped his huge hand back over mine and answered confidently, 'If it is, we'll deal with it. We've got through it before, we'll do it again.'

By the time we arrived home I had reconciled myself with the thought that until we knew the definite results of all the tests there was no point in me working myself up into a worried state over maybe's and what if's. I had a bit of a chat with God about it. I said, 'Okay Lord, if breast cancer is what you want me to go through, fine – I'll do it. But remember – I've got a rotten stinking temper and I'll fight that cancer. I won't let it ruin my life.'

That took a great deal of my worry away. The 'what if?' syndrome suddenly became a statement of 'what IS!'

I don't remember feeling any fear – apart from the initial shock of discovering the lump all those months earlier (which, incidentally, was based on zero diagnostic information). The thought of death did cross my mind, of course, but it didn't become the centre of my thinking. My main concern was focused on finding out the result, one way or another, so that I could get on with my life. To me, death was like the inevitable cold hard skin that forms on a warm custard, and that nobody likes. Once you peel off the yucky bit and put it in the bin you can gobble up the warm, sweet, rich splendour of the custardy pudding underneath.

Now I'm not one to brag about the size of my massive abundance of bosom, but, when I had the first series of mammograms, my 'girls' were too big for the machine. The Super K.X. # 17 dash 6 Model, reserved for us above-average buxom ladies, wasn't operating, so the radiographer had to take the X-ray of my breast in two parts and tape the pictures together. True!

They also needed two radiographers just to pick up my breast!

Just kidding.

Steve was allowed in with me during the breast ultrasound. He sat on a chair beside the bed while the sonographer drizzled cold blue lubricant gel on my right breast in a large double layered squiggly circle about five centimetres out from my nipple. As she finished it occurred to me that my bosom looked like it should have taken front row in the window of a fancy cake shop.

'My bosom looks just like a birthday cake!' I blurted out, laughing. At that moment my brain received the message from the nerves in my nipple that the gel was *cold*.

'With one candle!' I added proudly. My beloved just looked at the floor and shook his head in disbelief.

The specialist phoned me that Wednesday from hospital, between performing operations, to explain to me the results of all my tests. Gently he told me that I had cancer.

It sounds unbelievable, but at that very moment I felt no terror.

'Okaaay,' I replied slowly and calmly, while absorbing his words and accepting them. I felt no fear. Just a feeling of 'serene-ness'. I had been brought out of the darkness of the unknown, and now I knew what we were dealing with. Now I could fight it. 'Where do we go from here?'

He advised me that after an initial lumpectomy to remove the tumour ('mastectomy is not on the cards at this stage') I would have six weeks of chemotherapy, followed by six weeks of radiotherapy, then another six-week regime of chemo. He arranged a time for us to see him two days later so that he could explain everything in detail.

I rang Steve at his work to tell him. Then I sat down with our new puppy and cried. Not for the cancer, the possibility of death, or the word 'mastectomy', but for the impending loss of my beautiful naturally curly auburn–red hair to chemotherapy. I was upset over something as stupid as that – but not the stupid cancer.

I had such a strong desire that our lives continue with as much normality as possible – whatever the outcome. (Cancer is not a choice. Attitude is.) I love to laugh, and I wanted to keep on laughing in spite of having cancer. The way I figured the situation, I could sit on a chair in the corner of the lounge room and be bitter about it, or I could make the most of each day – enjoy life, retain my sense of humour and be better. Either way I'd still have cancer, but I decided the latter path required less effort. And I don't, by any stretch of the imagination, mean that I thought laughing and being positive would banish the cancer and make me get better physically. It's not about that. It's about being better psychologically. You can't help getting it: but you *can* help having it.

Steve and I sat down and had a chat about the situation with our two girls, then aged 8 and 6. We explained to them as much we could about the cancer and the expected procedure, chemotherapy and hair loss, in a way they would understand. We didn't want to bog them down with information overload, but we still wanted them to be as informed as possible – and involved as much, or as little, as they needed or wanted to be. (I didn't place any expectations on the way the girls 'should' cope. I understand that everyone deals with things in their own time and in their own way.)

I explained to them that there was a lump in my

breast that shouldn't be there (allowing them to feel it for themselves) and that I was going into hospital where a doctor would take the lump out.

Our oldest daughter Elissa, wiped away her tears and asked if I was going to die of cancer like the Grandma they'd never met (Steve's mum).

Kerrie, aged 6, was surprisingly excited about the whole thing. She planned to take the lump to school in a jar for 'Show and Tell'.

We spent some time talking with Elissa and Kerrie about the disease. In the end, like me, the thing that really upset them was the thought that mummy would have no hair.

They only began looking forward to the event when I told them they could put stick-on tattoos and draw texta pictures on my bald scalp to make it pretty!

The girls appeared to appreciate being part of a 'cancer treatment committee', and began coming up with all sorts of solutions; for example, a 'wig' made of coloured party streamers sticky-taped to my bald head.

I decided to keep them involved at the next step, so after their questions and our answers ran out I asked the girls whether there was anything they wanted Steve and me to ask the specialist on our next visit. We made a list.

Elissa wanted to know, 'What day will the operation be on? How long will Mummy be in hospital? Which hospital?'

Kerrie wanted to know, 'What food do they have?'

Sandy

My tumour grew at an unbelievable rate. At the time of diagnosis, it was already five centimetres in size!

The week before I went to see the doctor I was doing an intensive five-day course at work. Towards the end of that week I had noticed that my right breast was swelling. It was red, it felt hot, and the entire nipple area was drained of all colour.

I sat in one of the lectures towards the end of the week holding my bra-strap out from my chest because my boob was so sore.

During the initial examination the doctor suspected I had glandular fever. 'We'll do some tests and send them off for analysis straight away.'

He said the glands in my armpits and groin were so swollen it was glandular fever! That's what he said I had. Oh dear!

I struggled to put my bra back on. The doctor kept trying to convince me of his prognosis by saying, 'It's not your right breast *swelling*, it's your left one *shrinking*.'

'Don't be stupid!' I said. And with that, my bra-strap broke!

I said, 'Don't you think I should have a mammogram? There's something wrong!'

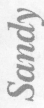
Sandy

That was when I *demanded* to have a mammogram.

Jim and I were given the news the following Monday. The mammogram had shown the breast was full of cancer. A biopsy was performed on my right breast in order to reveal just what type of cancer I had.

At the appointment after the biopsy a specialist suggested that a partial mastectomy be performed. Depending on the results of the pathology test taken during the partial mastectomy, it would be followed by a full mastectomy a few days later. This sounded like a lot of surgery for my poor old boob, so Jim and I decided that a second opinion was necessary before any operations were performed.

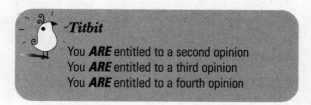

Titbit

You **ARE** entitled to a second opinion
You **ARE** entitled to a third opinion
You **ARE** entitled to a fourth opinion

I was referred to an oncologist (a doctor who specialises in tumours and prescribes adjuvant therapy). With the tiniest, gentlest soft hands, she felt all over my breasts and said, 'Sandy, the first thing we're *not* going to do is a mastectomy – we cannot touch that tumour!'

When we walked out of her door, Jim turned to me and said, 'She is going to save your life' – and she did!

The night Jim and I drove home from the doctor's surgery after we'd been given the diagnosis I made up my mind that this wasn't going to be the end of me! Cancer was just something I had to deal with, and then I would get on with life. We talked about it, we talked it over with the kids and here we still are, ten years down the track and looking fabulous!

I was so determined to keep living as normal a life as possible. I went in to work to see my boss the day after I'd been diagnosed. When I saw him and explained what the situation was I told him, 'You can put a For Rent sign on my chair – but you're certainly not putting a For Sale sign on it. I'm coming back to work!'

Diane

I found the lump myself.

Although I might forget to check for lumps the odd month here or there, I've always been fairly vigilant about self-examining my breasts. And it wasn't a classic 'lump' really. I felt what I would describe as a thickened area in my right breast. I checked my left breast. It also had a thickened area – though not as pronounced – in a similar position, so that in itself didn't alarm me terribly, but it did trigger me to investigate a little bit further.

I stood in front of a mirror and raised my arms up above my head to investigate any external changes. There was certainly a visible difference in the breasts. My left breast seemed slightly softer and smoother, but my right breast was more pronounced and seemed a little bit harder, with puckering of the skin. Immediately I thought, 'This is not good.'

I ended up booking an appointment for the following week (seeing that it was the earliest my husband Alan was able to have time off work to look after the children), but I figured a week wouldn't make much difference.

Diane

From the start I thought it was a breast cancer.

It wasn't a hasty analysis or what I wanted the outcome to be, and I certainly didn't wring my hands till they bled, thinking, 'It must be cancer; it must be cancer.' But that week's waiting period before I saw the doctor gave me time to reflect.

For the previous six months, but particularly for the three months before Christmas, I had been feeling like I was on an emotional roller coaster. I've always been a pre-menstrual sort of person, so I've had those waves of emotions, but I found myself experiencing a feeling of tiredness that I'd never had before. It had got to the stage where I would sit on the couch after dinner and be asleep within seconds.

In December I said to Alan that I thought I was 'losing it a bit'.

At the time I put it all down to the fact that I was a mother of three children and working two part-time jobs. I was also coordinating a number of end of year activities for the primary school – graduation dinners and so on. Our oldest son was completing his sixth year, so I was also doing the run around of secondary schools – just the usual things! *And* it was Christmas, so I thought, 'Diane, you're just pooped!'

But even though I thought I had the answer at the time I still wasn't comfortable with the way I felt.

After finding the lump it all made sense. I thought, 'This all ties in.' So I was fully expecting the doctor to tell me it was breast cancer, which is not like me at all.

Diane

On Wednesday morning I went to see my doctor. He felt the breast and agreed that it was a thickened area as opposed to a lump. But in Dr Bill's opinion, 'No lumps go uninvestigated.'

He told me there are only three ways he likes to treat a suspicious area in a woman's breast: mammogrammed, biopsied, or out! Dr Bill wrote out a referral for a mammogram and a second referral to see a specialist.

That afternoon I went off and had my mammogram. The radiographer said I could contact my doctor for the results at around five o'clock that evening.

When I phoned, Dr Bill had left, so I spoke to his colleague. I got the impression that she wasn't comfortable with the thought of dealing with me on the telephone, and that she would have preferred to speak with me at the surgery. She was very kind though.

She said, 'The results are back and they are highly suggestive of a breast cancer.' Had she said, 'I think you'd better come in and see me,' I definitely would have panicked. Then I'd have had to drive over there in a state of utter confusion.

I said, 'Okay, so "highly suggestive" means what?'

She answered, 'Well actually, when radiographers write reports, they're meticulously cautious in their diagnosis.'

Diane

I said, 'So "highly suggestive" then, is telling me that I have a breast cancer?'

'Yes, I believe so.'

'All right', I said. 'Where do we go from here?'

She told me that I still needed to see the specialist Dr Bill had referred me to.

I asked her what I needed to consider.

She said, 'I honestly believe you need to contemplate having a mastectomy. From what this report says, I think that's what they're going to suggest you do.'

So I was pretty well versed right from there. And because I'd already had a week to think about it before I saw the doctor I'd given it a bit of consideration anyway. I had started doing a little bit of investigating, so I knew roughly what kinds of options and procedures would be available.

My doctor's colleague turned out to be extremely helpful, and told me I could ring her at any time. She said, 'Any questions, day or night, I don't want you sitting on them. Just ask me.'

I finished the phone call. My legs went from under me. I had to force my legs to hold me up.

I had a tear, but I didn't *cry* cry. I sat down on the chair and all I could think was, 'Well this is all very well, but if worst comes to worst, who's going to look after my three children?'

I knew my husband would still be a wonderful father, but it's the impracticalities of him having to work as well as support a family. My thinking was taken over with, 'Who's going to look after my children during the day? Who's going to take them to school?

Who's going to do all those normal motherly things?'

I became consumed with the 'what if's'. What about my husband? What about my parents? What about my family?

It's strange, but what I was personally going to have to deal with really didn't come into play. My entire mind-set and the emotional impact of the news centred around thoughts of my family's predicament.

By this time, Alan had started his shift at work and I didn't feel I could phone him and tell him the results right at that moment. A short while later I'd thought of a few questions and rang my GP's colleague again. She reassured me with direct and open answers, which gave me a genuine feeling of support. (I think she was very smart. I think she allowed for the fact that sometimes when you're shocked you don't take in everything that's being said to you.)

I decided I wasn't going to cook tea that night and I wasn't going to cope with any mess, so I piled the kids into the car. We were going to have hamburgers.

The kids went outside to the playground while I stood in line to order our meals. When I got to the counter, and the girl said, 'Hello! How are you?' I opened my mouth to speak and simply dissolved into tears.

There I was standing at the counter of this busy restaurant crying, unable to speak and thinking, 'Oh, I don't believe this!'

The manager, Lindy, came over to find out what was wrong. She told the girl behind the counter to pour me a coffee, then turned to me and said, 'Come on Diane, let's go and find a seat.'

She sat with me as I blubbered out my story. She was sensational. She rounded up my boys, ordered their meals and delivered them to the table. She asked me if there was anything she could do. Did I need anything? Did I want her to drive us home? I think she did everything that anybody could ask for. And I only knew her from going into the restaurant frequently. Up until that day the extent of our conversation had been, 'Hello; how are you?' and 'Will that be dine in, or take-away?'

My kids ate their dinner and I pulled myself together. Then we went back home. All this time they didn't suspect anything was wrong. They'd been outside playing so they didn't see me fall apart. And because I'd been a bit emotional and teary for the past few months anyway it wasn't that uncommon for the boys to see me upset. They probably just thought, 'Uh ohh. Mum's got her period again!'

When we got home I walked up the road to see my friends Liz and Kevin.

Liz knew from my expression that something was wrong so she shuttled the boys out the back to play with her three girls. When the kids were out of earshot she turned to me and asked, 'What's wrong?'

I told her. She was an instant source of support and comfort.

Alan was still at work, but by this time I desperately wanted to go and tell him. Liz said I could leave the kids with her while I went to his office.

By the time I had driven the 45-minute trip to Alan's work I was quite composed. Al had no idea that I was coming in, so he was surprised to see me.

We went upstairs and I told him, 'I've had my mammogram and the results are not good. They're sure I've got a breast cancer and they're reasonably sure I'm going to have to have a mastectomy.' Just like that. Pa-bam!

And he said, 'Okay. Let's talk about this later. I'll just put my stuff away.'

His screen was up. I was taken aback. He wasn't responding to the news at all.

He took my hand and we went downstairs, got in the car and started driving home.

I thought that perhaps he hadn't understood me so I asked him, 'Are you aware of what I just said?'

'Yeah,' he answered casually. 'But you don't really

know anything yet. How can they know all that?'

I said, 'Because they've *told* me that's what it is!'

He just couldn't accept what I'd told him was fact. As far as Al was concerned it was still a case of, 'Well, they don't really know.'

Once we were home we talked more and he was so caring and concerned, but obviously in a state of disbelief. I think it was his way of coping. He was going to hang onto the hope that it wasn't 100 per cent proven.

That night I didn't sleep at all. The next night Al stayed awake all night to look after me and keep me company. This time I slept all night!

The following night (Thursday) we went to see the specialist Dr Bill had referred me to.

Dr Michael was extremely patient and spent about an hour with us. He was wonderful. His manner was calm, warm and humorous. My biggest issue that night was not being told about the breast cancer or the mastectomy; it was the thought of having to take my clothes off and get examined. I don't handle that well at all. Never have, never will. And it's got nothing to do with inhibitions. I couldn't care less about other people's nakedness, but my own offends me greatly. It's a fat issue; it's got nothing to do with anything else. That was my biggest problem at the time.

Having said that, Dr. Michael examined me as well

as anybody could have, and made me feel as comfortable as humanly possible.

He put the X-ray up to the light (which finally gave Alan and me a chance to see precisely what was going on within my breast) and said, 'That's not exactly what we want to see inside a breast.'

He was so patient and extremely reassuring, and answered all my questions. He explained everything about the surgery and the procedures to us, but added that he wouldn't be the man to do it. He said, 'My speciality is tummies, and Dr Richard's speciality is breasts. He's back from holidays on Monday, but we'll book you in to the hospital for surgery on Tuesday if you like.'

After I got dressed again I had more questions, 'So when will I meet this Dr Richard?'

'You'll meet him in hospital before you go into theatre. And he will certainly give you enough time to ask any questions you have for him.'

So I was pleased: I'd been given plenty of information about my situation and all my queries had been addressed.

Alan was still unconvinced about the whole thing. During the course of the conversation the doctor had said that when I did go into theatre a 'frozen section' would be performed. (The growth is removed, frozen, and sliced finely. The slices are then viewed under a microscope to ensure that the cancer is contained well within the boundaries of the area that has been cut out.) Until the frozen section had been examined there was no absolute way of knowing that I did in fact have cancer. But he did say he was 99 per cent certain that what he was looking at *was* a cancer; and that a mastectomy would need to be performed.

Still, there was that one per cent margin of doubt and that's what Alan latched on to. When we walked out of the doctor's office – even as I phoned my parents to let them know the latest up-dates – Al couldn't fully accept that it was cancer; he was still pretty much hoping it was a 'maybe'. He was coming *round* to the fact that it was cancer, and he was coming *round* to the fact that it would probably lead to a mastectomy, but he was still full of doubt – probably right up to the time I actually went into surgery.

I find it interesting that two people can be at the same doctor's appointment, hear the same words, and yet have two completely different interpretations of what's been said. I had *no* doubt in my mind, but then perhaps that's because it was actually happening to me, and I knew my own feelings and capabilities. I think with my husband it was an issue of protection. Men are naturally protectors of their families, and Alan is used to situations that come along that he can fix. He had no control over this; he couldn't fix it and he couldn't remove it. It was extremely threatening to him.

At this stage the kids had been given a rough outline of the situation, so now it was necessary to sit down and tell them exactly why I was going into hospital. At the time the boys were aged 12, 10 and 7.

I know with younger children there's a real death issue. Death is pretty terrifying. I explained that I had cancer in my breast and the way to get rid of the cancer was to have a mastectomy. Once you remove the breast or the tissue that the cancer is in you've removed the cancer – and it's all gone. They were all reasonably comfortable with that. The fact that I was telling them I was going to have my breast removed really wasn't an issue for them. The kids didn't really see the emotional impact of it.

And even though at the time, I'm sure deep down they felt threatened to some extent, they all seemed to deal with it fairly well.

Alan, my family and friends were all there for me – right from the start. I had wonderful support, love and the opportunity to talk and express how I was feeling. And it's amazing how much I relied on my sense of humour to get through it.

Doris

I encountered my first lump back in 1965. It was about the size and shape of a jellybean, and positioned near the nipple of my right breast. Because nobody talked about breast cancer in those days I ignored it. I just thought, 'That's a bit peculiar. I wonder what it is.'

It wasn't until 18 months later, when I went to see the doctor about another matter, that I said, 'By the way, I seem to have a jellybean stuck in my right boob.'

The doctor leaned over and fiddled with it, and said, 'Yes, you do.' She made an appointment for me to see a specialist the following day.

The specialist had a peek at my jellybean and mumbled, 'Mmm … hmm … hmm.' Then he left the room and sent a woman in, who booked me into the local private hospital the next morning. I asked her 'Does this mean I have cancer?'

And she said, 'Mmm … Mmm.'

Like I said; *nobody* talked about it.

> **Titbit**
>
> Write down any questions you want to ask your doctor. Some doctors permit the use of a tape recorder during the consultation, which is great because usually you forget the answers to your questions by the time you get home.

CHAPTER 3

Keeping a sense of tumour

(Accepting diagnosis)

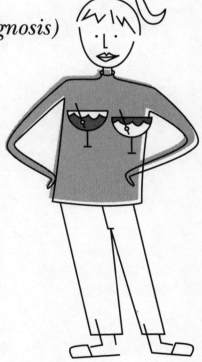

Gaye

My daughter's Grade 1 classroom was constantly unruly, which damaged her enthusiasm for taking articles to school for 'Show and Tell'. Instead of sitting quietly, many children would gather into small noisy groups, showing total indifference to the child at the front of the classroom.

The only time Kerrie was ever excited about 'Show and Tell' was the December when she told the class that I had breast cancer. She came home elated!

'Everybody listened, Mum!' she announced proudly. 'They all wanted to ask questions, and when I sat down on the carpet all the kids wanted to sit next to me and they were really interested, and they kept on asking me questions, even when it wasn't my turn any more! Then Shendy stood up to do her 'Show and Tell', but none of the kids listened to her because they were still talking to me. Then Shendy said that her mum had breast cancer too, so all the kids started listening to her as well!'

I laughed out loud at the joy I had obviously given my child. 'What sort of questions did the kids ask you, Kerrie?'

'Most of them asked, "What *is* breast cancer, anyway?"'

On Friday morning, as we got out of the car and walked across the carpark towards the surgeon's office, Steve stopped me and said, 'We'll go in and listen to what this bloke has to say, but if you don't like him that's it – we'll go somewhere else. You've got to be happy with him. With my brain tumour I got stuck with too many arrogant boffins – we're not going through that again and we don't have to put up with it. So if you don't like him, we'll just walk out and find someone else.'

The specialist ended up being absolutely marvellous. After telling his receptionists not to disturb us, he spent a leisurely 45 minutes explaining to Steve and myself about the cancer, the lumpectomy procedure and the removal of the lymph glands, and what to expect afterwards.

Still only wanting the best for me, Steve asked this gentle giant behind the big desk if he was the best bloke for the job. Rather than dazzling us with a speech about his eminence, he bashfully admitted that he and another doctor in the area just happened to be the specialists that the general practitioners this side of Melbourne tended to refer their patients to for breast problems.

Then I asked him with a sly grin, 'Is that because you're a good doctor – or do you just like looking at women's breasts?'

He stared at me speechlessly until we explained to him my philosophy of treating this cancer as an experience rather than an ordeal – and how important it was to me to keep a sense of humour.

He looked relieved, then let out a mighty laugh as he relaxed in his chair. He paused for a moment, then lent forward across the desk towards us and whispered with a cheeky, boyish smile, 'Well actually, I'll let you in on something ... When I came back from England 19 years ago I brought a new aspirator gun with me (the specialist-needled instrument used to drain the fluid from a cyst). All the GPs found out I had it and thought, "Gee, he must know what he's doing!" so they sent all their patients to me!'

As we sat in his office and laughed together, I realised he was much more than a doctor. He was a human being.

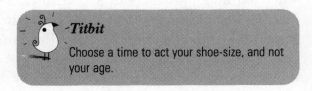

Titbit

Choose a time to act your shoe-size, and not your age.

It felt wonderful to be supported by such a hu-man. He kept us well informed without using patronising medical rhetoric or verbal flatulence. This man, with his penchant for trendy neck-ties and sports cars, still maintained the ability to reassure his patient, with a rich, velvety, deep voice like warm liquid chocolate that just makes you want to dive in and wallow, smothering yourself … and … huh? … where am I?

I shall call him Sir Galahad, for Galahad was a knight, pure and true (and he also carried around a great big cutty thing for making holes in people).

I must tell you, I originally considered naming him Dr Clark Kent, for the illustration of a superman concealed beneath the guise of an ordinary person, but I was worried that may have cast aspersions on his choice of intimate leg wear.

After our appointment with Sir Galahad, Steve and I intended to call in at my parents' house to let them know the up-dated details of the lumpectomy operation and hospital arrangements.

We stopped off first at our local bakery to pick up some morning tea. As well as buying a cake for the occasion I bought two golden, round, voluptuous, sugared doughnuts. Each one had a swirled blob of red jam on top – slap-bang in the middle.

Boosies in a paper bag.

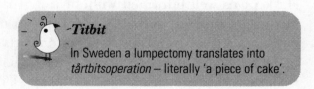

Titbit

In Sweden a lumpectomy translates into *tårtbitsoperation* – literally 'a piece of cake'.

Galahad explained the consequences of the axillary clearance (removal of the lymph glands from the armpit). If the cancer had spread to the rest of my body it would be evident in the lymph nodes.

Basically, the lymph glands sit in the armpit region and produce white blood cells and antibodies, which help defend the body against infection. The glands also act as a filter, preventing bacteria and harmful substances from flowing into the bloodstream. With the filter removed, the ability to fight infection is reduced.

I would be prone to lymphoedema (a condition of severe swelling that has no cure), so it was imperative to take extra precautions with that arm. Among the many preventative measures I had to avoid injury and strenuous activities such as heavy lifting and – wait for it – housework. Can you imagine how *that* grieved me? (See my likes and dislikes on the photo page!)

My blood pressure was to be taken and any

Titbit

Upon returning home, remember to maintain your arm-stretching exercises following lymph gland removal. I found a good exercise was to take the washing off the clothesline when it was dry. (I was fortunate to have a helper hang up the wet clothes.) Because it is quicker and easier to *remove* washing from the line my arms were raised for shorter amounts of time. It also meant that I didn't have to handle wet washing, which would have been too heavy for me to manage at that stage.

injections were to be given in the opposite arm. I had to avoid getting sunburnt, and wear rubber gloves while doing the dishes, gardening and so on.

I would also have to do special exercises after surgery to help recover movement and strength in the affected arm.

That afternoon I decided that if I couldn't use my right arm I'd make sure I could use the left. I implemented a similar strategy used by my great grandmother, after I remembered a story my grandmother had often told us.

My grandmother's older sister Violet contracted polio as a child, which resulted in her left arm being crippled. Their mother, determined that Violet should not become handicapped, but have a normal life like her sisters, constantly forced her to scrub the floorboards of the long hallway in their house with her left hand. My grandmother, Sylvie, remembered hearing her sister wail for hours while she laboured with a bucket and scrubbing brush until the job was completed. Violet had also confided in her that surely their mother mustn't really love her to act in so cruel a manner towards her already suffering daughter.

However, as time passed Violet's left arm developed greater strength than her right because of the regular exercise and massages her mother used to carry out on the tormented arm.

Violet grew up as active as any girl, and the disease did not prevent her from having the same prospects or life choices of any other young woman of her day.

My grandmother often testified, 'You wouldn't care

if she hit you with her right hand, but if Vi clobbered you with her left arm, you stayed clobbered – she could knock out a horse with her left fist!'

I decided that if it had worked for my Great Aunty Vi and it had worked for the Karate Kid in the movies (wax on ... wax off ...), surely it would work for me. I felt inspired and announced my plan to my family. However, due to the dog mysteriously developing a sudden and mysterious urge to bury every scrubbing brush that Steve brought home for me, I took the initiative and commandeered the kids' pole tennis. I began using it to improve the strength and co-ordination in my left arm and hand before and after surgery, and quickly became better at pole tennis with my left hand than with my right.

I was amazed at my newfound dexterity. I was able to make cups of tea, use the phone and the remote control for the television – all with incredible left-handed ease! Steve was equally amazed that my newly acquired ability did not appear to extend to dusting, filling up the washing machine, or unstacking the dishwasher, but like I explained, 'Who are we to question the powers of the totem tennis?'

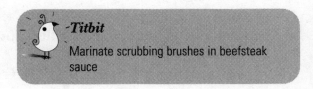

Titbit

Marinate scrubbing brushes in beefsteak sauce

Gaye

When Steve and I had seen Galahad that Friday morning he had booked me into hospital for the lumpectomy to be performed the following Monday. We had the rest of Friday and Saturday to run around and get things organised so that I could rest up on Sunday.

This was only 10 days before Christmas so my main priority was to get the kids' presents off various lay-bys, wrapped and hidden away, in the event that I wouldn't be up to it when I came home from hospital. As an excuse, I told the girls that I needed to go shopping to buy things for my hospital visit.

Because of this, the children's pre-arranged social plans took a back seat, much to the enormous disapproval of our youngest daughter, Kerrie. She was more than put out at the thought that we were going shopping for pretty nighties for mum, buying toiletries for mum – this for mum, that for mum. Everything for mum. We tried to explain to her many times that we needed to get everything done by Saturday so I could relax on Sunday, the day before the operation.

'_Well_ …,' she snarled, hands on her hips, mustering all the spiteful indignation possible for a girl of six. 'You just think you're the best, Mmmuuumm; _just_ because you've got _breast can-cer_!'

Steve and I looked at each other. His face echoed my frustration and hurt at her selfish insensitivity. I wanted to slap her.

But as we watched her march out of the room with her nose in the air I suddenly burst out laughing. I realised her concept of cancer was not that of a life-threatening disease – it was simply a great inconvenience.

I hugged her. I kissed her. *I learnt from her.*

Sandy

At the time of my first visit to the oncologist my eyesight was really bad. I couldn't even focus on the street directory to find where her rooms were. I was crying and working myself up into a real lather because I couldn't see on the map where on earth her practice was.

We finally found it and as soon as we emerged from our appointment Jim dragged me over to a public telephone and rang an optician. He said, 'Book in an appointment, I'm bringing my wife over and she's as blind as a bat. Give her some decent glasses!'

We drove down to the optician and while I was in there I thought to myself, 'I've got CANCER. Well! In that case I'm going to have Christian Dior glasses!'

I bought these great big super-expensive Christian Dior frames with diamantes on the side. I thought, 'If I'm going to die, I'll do it looking rich and absolutely gorgeous!'

Diane

Within the six-day period from when I had the mammogram to the day I went into hospital we'd let a lot of our friends know.

We had an enormous wave of support. We had friends just turn up on our doorstep with armfuls of food for the freezer, we had friends call in for a kiss and a hug. I had a wonderful circle of girlfriends from my kids' primary school who immediately pulled together with genuine offers of, 'We'll have the kids. We'll do the washing' and so on. 'Just one word and we'll be there.' And I knew that they would be.

One of our dearest friends, a policeman, happened to be at work when we phoned to tell him the news. Apparently he dissolved into tears and told his boss, 'I have to go and see a friend for a short while.' He drove straight over here in his police car, got out and just threw his arms around me.

Everybody was fantastic. It was really uplifting. I felt so buoyed by all the support I had. I went into hospital in the best possible circumstances. And yet at the same time, I knew that most of these people were coping well because I was coping well. It became pretty obvious early on – to most of the women I've spoken to, and certainly to myself – that as long as you're hanging in there, in control and feeling okay, your friends are feeling okay too. But it's a fine line. They'll accept a few tears; but if you drop your bundle completely, or you are in despair, they don't cope either. You can see that fragile link.

So the way people around you deal with your cancer depends a lot on your initial reaction and how you handle the issue for yourself. I wasn't setting myself up as a martyr; how I handled it was how I handle things normally. I didn't particularly set out to handle cancer any differently. It was just my natural response.

CHAPTER 4

A funny thing happened on the way to the theatre

(Surgery and hospital)

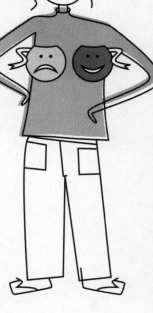

Gaye

Sir Galahad and Lady Kathy arrived at my bedside early Thursday morning with the results of the lumpectomy and lymph gland pathology findings. Fortunately, the lymph nodes were clear. The tissue removed from my armpit contained 18 lymph nodes. None of them showed signs of cancer involvement. This meant that the cancer was confined to my breast and hadn't wandered through into my blood system. However, there were extensive pre-cancers still living in my right breast.

We had no alternative and I needed no convincing. Complete removal of my right breast was the most pertinent solution. And as I was such a big girl bosom-wise, a reduction of the remaining left breast was initially advised, along with other surgical alternatives.

I quickly weighed up the information Galahad had empowered me with:

- A single breast would not allow me to make a comparison check if I found another lump or suspicious area.

- A single breast, reduced, would undoubtedly cause me to worry that a cancer might possibly be hiding behind the scar tissue and remain undetected during routine follow-up mammograms. I already knew what that felt like! (After Steve's brain tumour, which initially manifested itself as headaches, I worried every time he had another headache ... Had it come back? Had cancer cells escaped radiotherapy and started growing somewhere else in his brain? Is he telling me the truth about the severity of the pain because he doesn't want me to worry? – Just like he did two months after we were married, when he pretended to go to work but admitted himself to hospital because he knew by the type of pain that there was an associated problem.)

I didn't want to go through the wonder/worry stage again.

- A single breast, whether large or reduced would require a matching prosthesis – I definitely knew I didn't want to wear a prosthesis.

- A single breast, reduced, with a view to reconstructing a matching breast further down the track would annoy me: as a dressmaker, I prefer the 'clean slate' approach. I would rather create a complete new garment from scratch than fiddle around altering and matching bits and pieces from leftovers.

- A single breast, whether large or reduced, would not lower the 25 per cent chance of recurrence in the remaining breast. That's one in four – with those odds in a lottery you'd jump at the prospect of winning the payout! However, in this contest, first prize is the booby prize – cancer.

Weighing up all these options led to my big decision: total removal of both breasts.

I thought to myself, 'I'm comfortable with that!

I'm still woman; I'm still Gaye; I'm still alive.'

It made perfect sense to me to remove the environment that was playing host to such an insidious disease. Bilateral mastectomy (removal of both breasts) would eliminate that high chance of me maybe having to return to hospital in six months, or twelve months or two years, for the removal of the remaining breast due to recurrence. Less breast, less stress, *fewer needles*!

'Whip 'em both off at the same time,' I told Galahad. 'I'm attached to my breasts and they're very attached to me, but I'd rather worry about having no breasts than worry when the cancer was coming back.'

As I made my declaration I got the impression from Sir Galahad that he thought my decision and my acceptance of that decision had happened a bit too quickly. He said he understood that I had made my choice but he would give me a few days to think about it and then we'd talk again. However, I knew there was no way I would change my mind.

I phoned Steve from my hospital bed and told him the test results, the options and my verdict.

'I agree,' he said, unwavering. 'I think that's the best decision to make.'

Brimming with enthusiasm, I phoned my parents. Dad answered the phone. I relayed my conversation with Galahad and told him I'd be having a 'double whammy!'

He laughed. 'So you're going to look like Twiggy then?'

'Yeah, as flat as that!' I said laughing with him.

The happiness on his end of the line suddenly evaporated as he added solemnly, 'I don't know whether to believe you or not, Gaye.'

He couldn't be convinced. Here I was telling my father I would be to have both my breasts removed and sounding so happy about it! He put the receiver down and called my mother over to the phone.

During my stay in hospital some extremely kind mothers and children took it upon themselves to inform my 8-year-old daughter what to expect in relation to the surgical treatment of my cancer. 'Your Mum will have to have all her boobs *cut off* – but don't tell her, because she might get upset.'

Thank you so very much. NOT! This was the only time throughout the whole process that I became angry. The way I wanted to introduce my children to any degree of change had been taken away from my control; even more infuriating was the idea of expecting an 8-year-old child to carry this secret.

Fortunately though, I have a great relationship with my kids so we managed to keep any distress to a minimum.

Titbit

If you 'round down' people's two cents worth of useless information to the nearest zero, it becomes *nothing*!

During a visit with Sir Galahad before the operation I mentioned to him that during our discussion in hospital I had got the impression he had doubts about my decision to go ahead with the double mastectomy.

However, he said that he thought I had made the best choice. He just wanted to allow me some time for it to sink in.

I was also keen to find out how my chest would look post-op, with respect to the impending scars. Would it look like I'd slapped a couple of gigantic slices of Strassburg on my chest? How much of a cleavage would I own? Would I still be able to wear a revealing neckline?

I fired my concerns at this knight in shining armour and paraphrased it with one final question: 'When I look down, what will I see?'

He looked straight at me, deadpan, and said, 'Your feet!'

Gaye

While I felt sure that I had come to terms with, and accepted the news of, my cancer in the time it took me to acknowledge what Sir Galahad had told me over the phone, doubt began to creep in some weeks later. I began to think, 'Wait a minute; surely nobody can receive such disturbing news as cancer and accept it that quickly – then resolve to have a mastectomy without even batting an eyelash (Tinted: Charcoal-

Black # 04). Could I subconsciously be trapped in denial?'

Three months earlier my reaction to a diagnosis of cancer would definitely have been very different. Cancer, and death by cancer, had been a fear of mine. During those months I had been visiting a psychiatrist who had diagnosed me with major depression (an illness which I think is far more debilitating than cancer). He was in the process of helping me work through issues that had developed from unresolved childhood stuff. (There's enough material there for *Blue Buddies*, but that's another book!)

As with many people who have depression I had a chemical imbalance in my brain. It wasn't making enough serotonin – the body's natural 'feel-good' chemical.

At the time I was prescribed anti-depressants (suitable for my particular needs) to correct the chemical imbalance, and was learning to re-train my thought processes – from negatively based to positively based. It worked a treat! Little did I realise just how invaluable these new strategies would be in helping me to deal with such a fear head-on.

If I could get through cancer, then surely I could get through anything!

I explained the acceptance/denial quandary to my psychiatrist.

Gaye

From my diary:

I have been questioning myself as to how I feel. Every time I think intently about going into hospital on Monday for the mastectomy, my stomach starts doing weird things and I wonder whether my outward feelings are genuine or just a façade. I'm sick of having needles and that is honestly the most worrying aspect when I start concentrating on 'the next step.'

I accept that I have cancer and am assured of cure, but I wonder whether I have completed each of the five stages of grief: Denial, Anger, Bargaining, Depression and Acceptance. I feel that I have definitely reached the final stage of 'Acceptance', but I've skipped over all the rest. Did I complete the other stages while I was asleep, or am I coping extremely well using my newfound skills of logical and rational thought processes? I really don't like doubting this new confidence in my personal happiness and peace.

DENIAL: I have felt the tangible evidence of the lump. I have participated in many tests and have seen the two-dimensional evidence. I believe the prognosis of the doctor. But I feel, by the same token, physically removed from the cancer. I haven't been sick; I'm not jaundiced, and I'm still functioning as I did before I knew the lump was there. My mood hasn't changed; I'm still a happy person. I still joke around and instigate water fights with the kids in the street. It feels so surreal – internally and externally I feel wonderful – even with this cancer-thing inside me.

Only when I think intently about the situation do I worry that I'm subconsciously denying the disease (because I'm so well and continuing to go about the glorious business of living), but then when I cross-examine myself I don't see the sense in denying something when it's plain to see that it's there!

ANGER: I can honestly say I haven't felt anger towards any doctors, God or myself.

I don't give credence to the concept that I caused my own cancer or that I 'thought' it into being, as a number of today's self-attributing theories would have me believe. My great-grandmother died of a horrible cancer when my grandmother (Sylvie) was only 16 years old. From then on, Sylvie fully believed that any lump, bump, bruise or affliction she had was the result of a cancer; and that cancer would eventually be her cause of death. This was never fulfilled.

And I'm pretty sure that my Brownie Pack Leader, back in the mid '70s, had little medical evidence to support her fiery accusation to me, that 'If you keep biting your fingernails, Gaye – you'll get CANCER'. (I took my fingernails from my teeth and instead tried to bite back tears of fear. Then Brown Owl blew a long puff of elegant white cigarette smoke over us little girls and handed the glowing stub to her 7-year-old daughter to take outside the hall and throw into the garden.)

Over the years I've unconsciously done all the 'right' things, which are claimed to 'prevent' breast cancer. I eat pretty sensibly – I'm not overweight (I'm 175 cm tall, size 14 from the waist down – bust is 16E in a 'minimiser' bra). I breastfed my babies, am a non-smoker, an avid tea drinker, occasionally drink alcohol, I've never done illegal drugs, don't use underarm deodorant containing aluminium, I've had microwaved food about three times in my life and was on the (mini) pill for around ten minutes. And as for 'sexual repression' I'm definitely not a candidate ... but I'm not one to brag!

I don't believe this cancer is a 'punishment for sin', or for ringbarking Dad's apricot tree, or swinging round on the washing line after I was told not to. I do consider and have felt the whole episode to be a nuisance, as I am forced to put most of my activities on hold.

Some of my relatives have expressed anger and tried pinning the blame on one party or another. Probably because the lump wasn't picked up by the radiographer in the mammogram 20 months ago (which, in my personal case served as an advantage, because it gave me some time to learn and practise my new skills), or when I approached Dr Smith after I'd first felt the lump back in July (five months ago.) It was my decision not to have the 'cyst' drained, yet I don't blame myself. I knew (and know) in my heart and mind, that if Smithy had ordered me off for further testing after that first visit I would not have coped with the result. It's a double-edged sword.

As for Steve and me, there is no point in placing the blame on anyone. We don't need a scapegoat. I'm glad of the way the events unfolded, I know that I am now at a stage where I can look at situations and apply (to my mind) logical steps of accepting and appreciating the circumstances.

BARGAINING: This had not even entered my thinking! That's what pushes me to question whether I've arrived at the stage of Acceptance yet, even though I do feel a genuinely serene embracement of the situation.

I have thought along the lines of 'Was it because of the knock to my breast 15 years ago?' or 'Is it from excessive handling during foreplay and love-making?' But these are not the ploys of bargaining; they're what I would consider to be questions aimed at finding how the lump came about – which we invariably just won't know the answer to.

Therefore, I don't see the point in partaking of a bargaining exercise, which can't bring about a positive end for the amount of energy put into it!

DEPRESSION: See anti-depressant medication!

The anti-depressants don't deaden me to worrying influences; they merely supplement my body with the chemicals that my body isn't making enough of. It can be likened to a person with diabetes who requires insulin because their body isn't making enough of the chemical that their body needs.

The way I figure it – it's better to have two breasts removed because of cancer rather than two lungs due to it. At least I can still breathe a sigh of relief after surgery.

There's also the advantage of Steve having gone through cancer. (Yes, I *did* say advantage.) We have a rich communication and understanding with each other that helps tackle problems. And I'm still experiencing this incredible tangible source of comfort, which radiates out from my innermost being to every corner of my body.

ACCEPTANCE: We *have* been through cancer before, with Steve's Pinealoma and feel a bit like we've 'been there, done that'. I think that if we didn't have that experience to draw on I would be taking things a little more seriously. We know God is with us, and we'll get through it!

We are treating this cancer as an experience – not an ordeal.

When I had finished, my psychiatrist assured me that the five stages of grief were not compulsory. It is indeed possible to move straight to acceptance, as I had done.

Just before they came to take me to theatre for the mastectomy, Steve and I prayed together. (What does one pray at a time like this?! 'As I lay me down to sleep?' 'For what we are about to receive may we be truly thankful. Amen?' Yeah, the same one I say when I dive into the oogly-moogly end of the waterbed with my soul mate!)

Then he kissed me. Next he kissed gently each beautiful bosom that adorned my body, and that had comforted my lover and fed our babies. Then he kissed me again on the mouth. A long sweet kiss. This did not feel like a sad event – the passing of my breasts. I knew it was the best thing for me to do.

After I was wheeled into the operating theatre for the bilateral mastectomy, I asked the theatre sister for a piece of surgical tape and a pen. I wrote 'B O O B!' in large letters on the tape, then crossed out the last 'B'.

Now it read 'B O O !' Sticking the message over the lumpectomy scar on my right breast, I covered up and waited to go to sleep.

Back in my room, as soon as I was able I rummaged under the bandages and padding to view the handiwork of my knight of the stainless steel table. I had expected a single line spanning the width of my chest, but I stared in awe at two separate lines where each breast used to be and softly said to myself, 'You wonderful beautiful man, you gave me a cleavage!'

The following morning, Sir Galahad came in to check on my progress. He opened up the conversation by saying 'Boo!'

'So you got my message then?' I enquired.

'We all cracked up,' he grinned. 'We laughed so much we couldn't operate for a while!'

THE TOP 10 REASONS

FOR HAVING A MASTECTOMY

10 No one can accidentally park their bicycle in your cleavage.

9 On a cold day, your nipples won't get caught in the closing doors of a lift.

8 You know when your shoes need cleaning.

7 Your nipples won't need to be consulted to determine the outside sub-zero temperature.

6 You won't be disqualified for touching the wrong coloured spot with a dangling body part while playing 'Twister'.

5 You won't be disqualified for touching the wrong spot with a bouncing body part while playing hopscotch.

4 You'll never again have a bra the same colour as dryer lint.

3 Your boobs won't accidentally get tucked into your jeans with your shirt.

2 Your chest will no longer reverberate for three minutes after you stop jogging or using a skipping rope.

1 And the number **ONE** reason for having a mastectomy … That the spring in your step when you walk is caused by knowing you have done all you could to stay alive.

Sandy

It turned out that I had a rare form of breast cancer that was particularly aggressive. At that point in time – and in my case – a mastectomy was out of the question.

A regime of six treatments of chemotherapy (one a month) and 30 lots of radiotherapy would be followed by an iridium implant. Now, at this point I didn't know what an iridium implant was from a tree growing in the backyard, and I was going to have it two weeks after my final hit of radiation!

It turned out that the treatment consisted of long knitting-needle type rods to be inserted into my breast while I was under a general anaesthetic. There were 18 rods in total, each one about 12 inches long. Each one went in through one side of my breast and came out the other side. These were then plugged into a machine that delivered radiation straight into the tumour. I had to be wired up for 72 consecutive hours. Three days and nights of constant radiation.

I was put in a bed in an isolation ward. A solid lead shield was set up across the doorway. It was three inches thick and came up about three-quarters of the way up the door.

Jim and my daughter, Sharon, used to come and visit me but they had to stand outside my room. They weren't allowed to come in because of the constant radiation. I felt like a chook in a fowl shed with all these people peering over the top of the lead shield at me!

The controls and all the switches were on a wall outside the room. The only time anyone could come near me was when I needed to use the toilet. When I needed to go, the implant would be turned off, then they could enter the room and unhook this thing. Then, while one nurse was taking my blood pressure, another nurse would take my pulse. Someone would give me a wash, someone would shove my dinner under my nose, someone would bring fresh water and someone else would make the bed, all in a matter of minutes. These changes had to take place quickly because they wasted time.

After a short rest at home following the implant I was told it would be necessary to have another six months of chemo – followed by a mandatory long holiday to recover!

Diane

Tuesday morning I went into hospital. While I was being booked in I noticed the most magnificent bouquet of tiny yellow rosebuds sitting on the reception desk. I turned to Alan and whispered, 'Aren't they gorgeous!'

The Admitting Nurse noticed my name and said, 'Oh, those flowers are for you!' The principal from the school had sent them along with a small note. I don't think anything has affected me as much as that gesture. The roses came down to my room with me, so I had flowers before I'd even had an operation. I thought it was just amazing.

A lass who introduced herself as Marlee picked us up from reception. She said, 'I'm in charge of paediatrics. I'll take you to your room.'

We began walking down the corridor to the paediatric ward, when her words suddenly struck me. My grip tightened on Alan's hand. I thought '*Paediatrics*? What on earth would a paediatric nurse know about a woman having a mastectomy? What do they know about boobs? I'm not a 7-year-old having my appendix out! Paediatrics for goodness sake?!'

We stopped at a private room. Marlee settled me in (she was lovely). She said, 'Don't worry about getting changed. At this stage you're welcome to watch the telly, read a book ...'

'... Play with Lego?' I wondered.

(I needn't have worried. We were told later on that they occasionally have adults in the paediatric ward due to the number of private rooms. And I soon learnt how marvellously supportive, compassionate and understanding the paediatric nurses were.)

Theatre was booked for two o'clock and as the morning melted into lunchtime I started feeling really toey. I was agitated because I still hadn't met the surgeon who, I believed, was going to remove my breast. Also I was anxious because of that body issue again. I had to get undressed once more – and I realised that underneath my dress I wasn't prepared! (If I have to go to the doctor to have any area examined I'll wear a skirt or trousers – because I only want to take off the minimum amount of clothing.)

I could hear the words of my mother, 'Yes Diane, always wear a petticoat.'

This was beginning to feel really ugly. I knew the doctor would come in and say, 'Let's just have a look before you go to theatre!'

We heard a gentle knock on the door. Al opened it to find my cousin Wendy and her daughter Jody. An unexpected visit – and just what I needed to take my mind off my horrors.

At about one o'clock the surgeon, Dr Richard, turned up. He gave me all the facts again and went over the procedure. I asked him if he was 'neat'. I said, 'I know this isn't going to look brilliant, but I really want neat.'

'Yes, I'm neat.' He assured me.

I said, 'Yes – but are you *very* neat?'

As I waited in the pre-op area Al was able to stay with me. He sat there talking, holding my hand, stroking my forehead – anything he could do he did – and I went into 'babbling overdrive'. Saying things like, 'Give me one more cuddle, because no one will want to cuddle me after today, because they'll feel I have only one breast.'

I was wheeled into theatre and poor Al was left alone to wait and mull over my pre-op ramblings.

In the theatre room a gorgeous man walked up to me, held my hand, and explained, 'I've just got to get you ready and put a few sticky things on you. But for the rest of the time, until you're asleep, I'm here holding your hand and I'm not going to leave you for a minute.' He placed his other hand on my shoulder – and a greater comfort I've never known.

The anaesthetist was having trouble finding a vein, so I kept chatting to Mr Gorgeous to keep my mind off it. We talked about the photograph on the ceiling, which had a group of masked surgeons peering down over the operating table. He also explained the 50 dollar note pinned to the ceiling directly above us.

'If you're still awake by the time you get to the number they want you to count to, you get the money!' (It stays there – trust me. That 50 dollar note has been there a long time.)

The anaesthetist still hadn't found a vein, and I was beginning to think, 'I'm going to lose it.'

All of a sudden I could feel the tears welling up,

and I turned to him and said, 'Do you think you could give me something to get me to sleep and do that afterwards, cos otherwise I'm not going to cope.'

He said, 'Not a problem.' And that's the last thing I knew.

Alan waited at the hospital throughout the operation and as soon as it was possible he came and sat by my bedside. He sat there for hours just stroking my head. I felt the most amazing love and support from Al. I could see it. I could feel it. He *was* there for me all that time.

And while I knew my husband loved me, and I thought knew me fairly well, over the course of following days and months ahead I found out that he loved me even more than I had ever imagined, and seemed at times, to know me better than I even knew myself.

When I woke up properly the first thing I can remember doing was putting my hand on my chest. I thought, 'Yep! It's gone.' That didn't overly phase me; I had expected my boob to be gone.

Even though in some respects it was a stressful period, I had a brilliant time in hospital. I had magnificent nursing care and outstanding doctor support. Dr Richard was considerate and empathetic – just lovely – which gave me great confidence in him. Alan, Mum and Dad, my sister and brother in law, my whole family and all our friends were there for me. I had 100 per cent support. I felt wholly loved.

Doris

At eight o'clock in the morning, as instructed, I was in the hospital, wearing one of their lovely white, starched frocks with bows down the back. By lunchtime the breast had gone.

When I came round from the surgery, all stuck together with sticking plaster, a nursing sister said, 'You're perfectly all right. You're in hospital and your breast has been removed. It's all gone very well.'

I remember thinking, 'How marvellous. It didn't take long at all.'

I wasn't shocked that the breast had gone because one of the nursing staff had told me what the procedure would be: the doctor would remove the lump, check it and if it was cancerous the breast would be removed.

At that time I had my mother and my two children living with me. I hadn't told my mother anything about it. I just said I was having a test (or something silly). One of my bosses ended up with the responsibility of going to the house and telling my mother what I was actually in hospital for.

> **Titbit**
>
> If you have had lymph glands removed from under your arms, you will find a deodorant spray will feel kinder to your armpit than the pressure and sensation felt when using a roll-on deodorant.

CHAPTER 5

Bouncing back

(Post-operative)

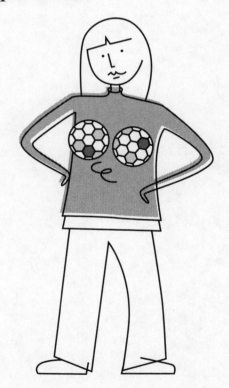

Gaye

The day after the mastectomy I 'ran a book', getting family, friends and visitors to guess the weight of my extracted bosoms. My sister Ros had the closest guess at 'four kilograms'. My beloved's estimate didn't count – he cheated and got a nursing sister to check the pathology report.

(The pathology report also revealed that under close examination my left breast – my *good* breast – contained 'occasional cysts' throughout the tissue. Though they showed evidence of 'change' they were not malignant. And while the changes were detected without the use of a microscope they had not been identified in my mammograms. Scary!

I already knew that I'd made the right decision in removing both breasts – knowing *myself* and my capabilities – this news was just further reinforcement that I'd chosen the best option.)

I also decided to get my visitors, and the wonderful nursing staff who were involved with the mastectomy, to sign my last bra as a 'fitting mamm-ento' – not that it would ever be fitting me again, but I think you know what I mean. I thought, 'If I were here in hospital with a broken arm or leg, I'd be getting people to sign my plaster cast, so why not my bra?'

The majority of those I asked were delighted with the unprecedented request. Others were visibly overwhelmed but agreed to comply with the mad cancer girl, then hurried out of the room. Eventually

Gaye

I framed it, padded out the cups, and hung it on our lounge-room wall.

Gaye's 'Wonder Bra' Messages

Sweet Mammaries are made of this

Best Wishes – *Margaret*

To Wonder Woman, the sexiest flat-chested woman we know

Hang in there

Best Wishes – *Jenny*

Gaye, Your provac remover – Take care, *Sue W.* (Provacs are the drainage bottles.)

Liss your Loveing girl

Shoulders will feel lighter

I have always envied women who are bra-less

Wishing you all the best. *A. Smith*

D. Pratt

June may be busting out all over, but not Gaye any more!

Best of luck with the new set!

Best Wishes, *Sheila*

KERRIE ♥

To my Darling Big Sis, you will always be way out in front to me.

Welcome to the IBTC (the Itty Bitty Titty Committee!)

This was too much bosom for any one woman. XXX

And my most favouritist ones ...

Dearest ♥ Gaye ♥ You're simply the breast.

Dear Gaye, Boo! to a very brave girl. – *Sir Galahad*

You're all heart
MUM ♥

(After Mum wrote her message, she leant over and whispered to me, 'I wrote mine there, because that's where your bra was laying over your heart.)

On the third day after my mastectomy, the metal staples had to come out. All 79 of them. I was told it would hurt. Rhonda, the nursing sister who drew the short straw, brought in a staple remover and a 44 gallon kidney dish for the shrapnel.

Now there wasn't much feeling in my post-breastal region, so I reckon it hurt her more, particularly as I wasn't watching. After about the seventh staple along my giant steel zipper and having counted the number of ceiling panels twice, I looked at Rhonda's face. Every now and then a staple being removed would get stuck in my flesh and she would wince empathetically, 'ooh-ing' and 'argh-ing.'

I said to her, 'Rhonda, you're not supposed to say "ooh" and "argh" like that. It makes the patient think something's wrong. Do what a hairdresser does when they make a mistake while they're cutting hair. They don't say "ooh" and "argh", they just say "There we go-o-o-o!"'

From then on she took my advice, so 58 more times she said, 'There we go-o-o-o!'

Although I loved my time with the tremendously supportive nursing staff (I still call them my angels – because that's what they were!), by Friday I was getting excited at the prospect of going home again. And although I desperately wanted to be back home, Steve and my Mum were worried that if left alone I might misbehave and, perhaps –

- spring-clean the house. (Oooh yuk, I would never do that!)

or

- maybe take part in a game of neighbourhood cricket. (ka-BOOM!)

They plotted between themselves that after Steve picked me up from hospital, he would drop me off at

Mum's and return to work. Mum kindly decided I should be kept suitably busy (in a restrained sort of way) and took me off to a shopping centre for a bit of fiscal therapy – her shout.

Mum said, 'Gaye, if you're too sick to go clothes shopping, then you're *really* too sick!'

(I was wearing the dress that I'd worn to the hospital when I had bosoms. The day I went in, the princess-line design and soft fabric draped delicately over my supple breasts, tucking slightly in at the waist, gliding over my abdomen to hide my mother tummy. The day I came out, the fabric of my dress drifted over barren plains where the enemy had once hidden, tucking in slightly at the waist and ricocheting a fine cotton polyester blend – at full shrapnel force – over and around my, now more obvious, belly of plenitude.)

We weren't in the shopping centre five minutes when Mum met a friend she hadn't seen for a few years. Mum introduced me to her friend, who politely responded with 'hello', then noticed my tummy and asked sincerely, 'And when are you due?'

I laughed and told her I'd just come out of hospital, and that I'd had a mastectomy four days ago.

We revived the lady (with a gleaming pair of defibrillators I just happened to have in my handbag; CLEAR – 360 – STAT!) and she apologised for offending me.

I definitely wasn't offended, though I decided that jeans and tee-shirts might be a good way of harnessing my podge. (I also found the short baby-doll style dresses were another excellent alternative. The gathering sits at the bust area so that the lack of breast isn't readily noticeable and billows out to hide the tummy area.)

About a week after the mastectomy, Elissa and I were having a cuddle. She gently (very gently!) rested the side of her head on my flat chest for a moment, then pulled away suddenly staring at me in astonishment. 'Mummy!' she squealed with delight. 'Now I can hear your heart beating'!

Weeks after the mastectomy, I saw a friend from school at the swimming centre. I told her it was the first time I had gone swimming since the operation. She looked down towards my flat chest under my bathers, then back at my face. Slightly puzzled she asked seriously, 'Will you still be able to float?'

Speaking of swimming, admittedly I did have a bit of trouble with breaststroke after the mastectomy – but now I just use my arms like everyone else!

Sandy

The cancer and treatment didn't stop us from doing anything. We went to the kid's social functions at school, we entertained at home and we continued to go out for dinner. (We would sit in the restaurant and play 'pick the wig'!)

Diane

Alan sat down with the boys while I was in hospital and gave them the details about the operation so that they weren't upset or mortified by it all. Soon after I returned home my two youngest children, Matthew and Phillip, asked me, 'Can we have a look at your scar?'

I said, 'Of course you can' (though secretly I was dreading that moment).

I knew that they were interested in a big cut and lots of stitches because that's the impressive bit. Phillip, the youngest, was quite impressed (although there could have been more stitches). But because it was big and it looked pretty angry he was satisfied.

The boys were not in the least bit disturbed or

horrified by my chest (which I thought was a good sign). They sat back down on the floor playing with their toys and chatting about my mastectomy wound. Suddenly one of the boys stopped what he was doing and looked back at me and asked, 'Mum, when will your bosom grow back again?'

During the time after I first came home from hospital, I became acutely aware that for some people it was very difficult to look me in the face. Their eyes would focus on my chest. I think they were trying to work out, 'Which breast has she had off?'

I noticed it most at the school. Just about everyone in the school community had heard about my mastectomy. And that in itself didn't bother me, but I found it rather daunting the first few times I went back up to the school because I knew that I was the focus of people's attention. A number of times, while talking to people, I found myself bending at the knees to meet their eye level. They seemed so fixated on talking to my boob and prosthesis, that they weren't even looking me in the face.

In the end it got the better of me. I was in the canteen with a group of girlfriends when I announced, 'Tomorrow I'm going to wear a sticky label with an arrow on it saying, "IT'S THIS ONE!"' We had a giggle, made the sign right there and then in the school canteen and pinned it on my tee-shirt.

Doris

There was an old woman in the bed next to me.
Actually, she was younger than the age I am now!

I'd had my right breast removed, and she, her left.
I organised the beds around so that we could be 'book
ends'.

It was after the departure of my first boob that I met
Richard, my second husband. (Actually, I had met him
before that, but he hadn't become intimately
acquainted with my breasts at that point.) We were
friends and I had been keeping him informed about
what was going on. When the friendship suddenly
developed into something more, I said to Richard,
'Do you mind terribly ... ?' (He was inexperienced
with women you see, but he had no worries about the
number of breasts that I owned. He was marvellous
about the whole thing. He thought single-breasted
wives were as fashionable as his double-breasted suits!)

He was lovely. And I think, at the time, one breast
was probably more than enough for him. The poor
man wouldn't have known what to do with two!

Twenty-three years later when I found a lump in my remaining breast, it was a bit more alarming. This time it was extremely big, and sitting close to my sternum.

The mammogram was pretty conclusive. Cancer. It looked to me like a great big flat hamburger patty. I named it 'Mack'. Fortunately though, it hadn't metastasised (spread). It hadn't set off on a great journey though my body, but a mastectomy was unavoidable.

By now, the surgeon had become a personal friend. (I fell madly in love with him.) And the day 'arrived'. I was doped up, wearing my lovely white frock again, but the operation was unexpectedly called off. The surgeon had been involved with surgery the night before, which had gone on much longer than anticipated, so all his morning operations were rescheduled to the following day.

He came to see me in the evening of the day on which I was supposed to have been 'done', carrying a single rose, which he presented to me with a flourish. (Mind you, he'd stolen it from the hospital rose garden, but that was a moment where I thought, 'How lovely.')

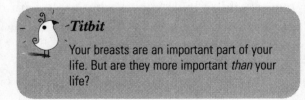

Titbit

Your breasts are an important part of your life. But are they more important *than* your life?

CHAPTER 6

Cysters are doing it for themselves

(Self-examination)

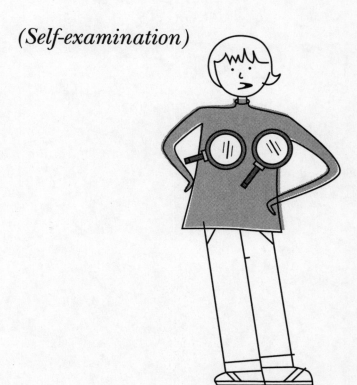

Gaye

Because breast cancer is the most common cancer in women, and it doesn't always indicate its presence by obvious accompanying illness, it can't be stressed enough that early detection and treatment is fundamental for a successful outcome.

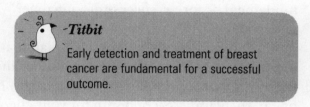

Titbit

Early detection and treatment of breast cancer are fundamental for a successful outcome.

It has been recommended that women should start practising self-examination at age 35. That's fine, but I was 32 when I found my lump and the tumour had been alive and kicking inside me for over two years before that, and there was no family history of breast cancer!

I regard myself as having been spoilt by the fortune of having a caring GP who listens to his patients' concerns, takes all things into consideration and then explains everything in simple terms. I know he believes that women are potential hosts for this disease regardless of their age.

Please don't be persuaded not to check your breasts because you are statistically 'too young' for breast cancer, or your breasts are 'too fibrous' or you are told, 'No, it's not necessary; they're lumpy because you're breast-feeding.' (The number of women who are diagnosed while still breast-feeding amazes me.) If you have any concerns, see your doctor. If you feel you're not being heard, talk louder. Remember the titbit: You *are* entitled to a second opinion.

And remember how I said it can't be stressed enough that 'early detection and treatment is fundamental for a successful outcome?' Well I'm saying it again!

The best time for a routine examination each month is a few days after your period has finished. In the event that you no longer have periods, decide on one particular day each month for your check. A great place to do this is in a relaxing, deep, mineral salt bath or bubble bath. Wait till the kids are asleep (the less distractions the better), take in your favourite drink and music, maybe some candles for soft light. Make an occasion of it!

If you are able, tilt or lie backwards and go over each breast with a soapy hand. This enables smoother contact so that changes close to the breast surface can be identified more easily. Use the Anti-Cancer Council guidelines to examine deeper into the surrounding tissue. Repeat this procedure while sitting, as the breast will respond differently when you change position. The same can be performed while you are in the shower (standing up obviously).

Before you leave the bathroom, do a mirror check on the external appearance of your breasts, and when you retire to bed fully go over each breast again while lying on your back, taking full advantage of being able to examine your breasts while they are resting in yet another position.

Recording the dates and any changes or suspicious areas on a diagram will help you to remember variations from the month before. These will either alleviate any worry or give you a background to present to your doctor!

The number of younger women diagnosed with breast cancer seems to be increasing. A doctor told me of two separate cases where the women were both aged 22 at the time of their diagnosis.

As a woman who has had breast cancer I would like to suggest beginning self-examination as early as 16 years old. I don't want to instill fear or use scare tactics, but at least it will get you into some sort of regular practice for the rest of your life, and you will become familiar with the layout, structure and characteristics of your breasts. Getting used to your breasts – knowing them – makes most changes easier to detect.

I remember an awareness campaign when I was younger that suggested taking a small piece of cotton wool, rolling it up to the size of a pea, and placing it between your bra and breast. Passing your fingers across your bra and over the lump of cotton wool simulated how a possible lump or cancer would feel.

Over the years of self-examination, I hunted for that soft pea-sized lump, obviously hoping never to find it, which is probably one of the reasons for my initial anxiety when I found a lump the size of a brazil nut.

Women need to be reminded that there is no one singular way of presenting with a lump. That's why anything unusual or suspicious should be professionally checked. Remember that nine out of ten lumps are non-threatening and early detection is the best advantage for a successful outcome.

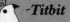

Titbit

Remember ... if you keep on top of your breasts, they should keep on top of you. Early detection and treatment is fundamental for a successful outcome.

CHAPTER 7

A girl's breast friend

(Gift ideas)

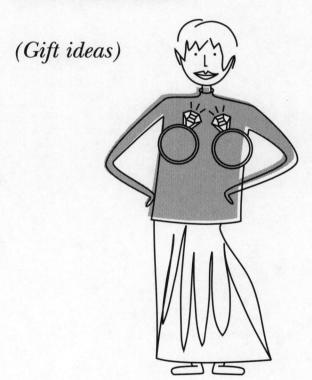

Gaye

These are just some of the many wonderful and helpful items and household hints I appreciated during the initial period of diagnosis and hospitalisation.

Loofah gloves

I ended up buying four pairs of these, I loved them that much, and I still use them every day. They are made from rough synthetic yarn, knitted into gloves and are worn while bathing or showering. They're great every day, but especially useful after surgery when you don't want the heaviness of a wet flannel on tender skin. The rough texture stimulates nerve endings, which is wonderfully invigorating. (If using them in hospital following surgery, I'd suggest packing more than one pair so that you have a clean pair – for hygiene reasons – each day.)

Journal

Some years ago, during a rare bout of spring-cleaning, I rediscovered a small notebook hidden away among some books in a storage box. It belonged to Steve and dated back to 1985 when he was diagnosed with a cancerous tumour on the pineal gland. He had used this notebook during his time in hospital to jot down conversations between specialists and himself, note reminders to himself of questions he wanted to ask doctors, and occasionally record his own observations.

Sometimes, if he was sleeping when I came to visit, or he had not yet returned from an operation, I would write a message for him to find.

This notebook was a poignant reminder of those frightening times but it also served as an important milestone because we have travelled such a long way together since then. (I remember when I found this notebook and flicked though each page absorbing the daunting memories, I regretted that there was such a small amount of recorded information in proportion to the events that were taking place during that time. And as I replaced the notebook in its box I thought flippantly, 'Boy, if I ever had cancer I'd write a whole *book.*'

Writing down your thoughts (even if nobody else reads them) can be a great personal outlet. And it may not be until much later that you appreciate the fact that those thoughts have actually been recorded. An elegant notebook set aside for this purpose lends a special feeling of importance to the situation.

From day one I was grateful to be able to see so many advantages within my cancer incident. If my spirit flagged I would look about and search for an extra special positive experience to brighten my day (not necessarily relating to cancer). These were often just simple things such as secretly watching a magpie wandering about the garden collecting materials for its nest, or my night walks – where I could see the awesome beauty of the stars and moon. I would note these profound moments in my journal. Ordinarily, these occurrences don't seem particularly exciting but when I looked at them through the renewed eyes, heart and mind of a cancer patient, 'small things' became great!

I think that once you do start searching for positive thoughts, words from a song or observations, it becomes easier to see them more often. If, in your personal situation, you can find just three things daily for which you can be grateful, or which made you feel happy or special, write them down in your journal. They'll be waiting there for you next time you need a quick pick-me-up.

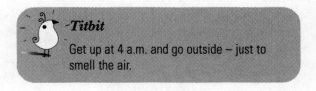

Titbit

Get up at 4 a.m. and go outside – just to smell the air.

Massage

A professional massage is wonderful at the best of times. How much better can it be at the worst of times?

(I have since found the most wonderful massage therapist, who is also able to redirect built-up lymphatic fluid in my right arm – my lymphoedema arm – after I've become too active for my own good.)

When using the services of a massage therapist, ensure that they are fully trained and qualified, and registered with an accredited association.

Candlelit bath

This is a luxury for anyone! Run a deep, mineral salt bath or bubble bath. Light some candles so you can relax under soft lighting, select some soothing music to listen to (keep the stereo or tape player well away from the water), grab a drink, a magazine or book and just soak for at least 30 minutes.

Fruit loaf

During chemo and radiation therapies, particular drugs have a tendency to 'bind you up'. I know a cancer lady who looked forward to this weekly cake, made by a good friend.

Joanie's fruit loaf
1 cup Allbran
1½ cups dried fruit
1 very ripe banana (mashed)
1 cup milk
1 cup self-raising flour
½ cup sugar
½ teaspoon mixed spice

Method
Soak the Allbran, dried fruit, mashed banana and milk for 1 hour. Mix in the flour, sugar and spice until combined. Pour mixture into greased loaf pan. Bake in moderate oven (180°C) for 35 minutes.

To microwave
Pour mixture into microwave loaf pan. Cook on medi-

um heat for 12–15 minutes. Leave in microwave oven for 5 minutes before removing from pan.

Breast Cancer Action Nova Scotia (bcans)

www.bcans.org

Click onto the 'main discussion forum' or the 'Off Topic' for 'not so cancerous' subjects. An informative and supportive Internet forum for breast cancer people, their family and carers. (This is the best and most up-to-date site that I've found.)

Help from the family

Steve, Elissa, Kerrie and my extended family were terrific with help and support. The washing was done, the clothes were dried, folded and taken away in washing baskets and returned – all beautifully ironed. When I got a bit stronger I wanted to try and do stuff around the house without having to constantly rely on Steve or the girls dropping what they were doing to assist me. I worked out new methods so I could do everyday tasks.

In the kitchen

Kitchen-wise I've always adored the joys and synergy of cooking, food preparation and presentation. During my recovery I found it much easier to cook one-pot meals such as risotto, pasta dishes and casseroles. The stirring was possible with my left arm, without putting a strain on my right, and I just got everyone to dish up their own portions.

Two great purchases were a wok, which enabled tasty one-pot cooking, and a mandoline. The mandoline allowed me to cut and slice vegetables evenly. I could hold the vegetables in my right hand (it felt far too dangerous to do it with my left) and slide the veggies across the mandoline's blade without the jarring action associated with a chopping knife.

My poor little mortar and pestle have had limited use due to the extra stress the pounding action puts on my right arm, so I've had to make do with a grinding action pepper mill for peppercorns and an inexpensive coffee mill picked up from the supermarket (with metal grinding components and wooden casing) for my whole spices, such as cloves and allspice for cake-baking. Both mills can be operated using either hand.

I tried as much as possible to 'lead with my left hand', though if it felt too awkward or dangerous I usually tried to find an alternative method before resorting to using (and injuring) my right arm. Take, for example, mashing potatoes – now there was a lesson in uncoordination and how to get a messy stovetop! I soon found that an inexpensive, small hand-held, electric food mixer (used in either hand) did the trick much better, mixing and whipping up those potatoes into a thick, creamy, velvety-white mash.

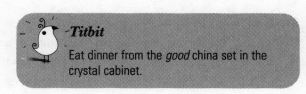

My girlfriend Jess gave me a gorgeous tasting 'slice recipe' that was prepared and mixed in a saucepan! Unable to eat 'a slice', I ended up transforming it into cakes and/or muffins (using a metal, swivel-action, ice-cream scooper in my left hand to deliver even amounts of the cake mixture to the muffin tray. I also bought a smaller scooper, available from specialty kitchen shops, which was a perfect size for biscuits.)

Dana's raisin slice (Jess's mum)

1 cup chopped raisins
1 cup water
125 grams butter (or margarine)
1¾ cups plain flour (I actually use 1 cup of stone-ground wholemeal flour and ¾ cup plain flour)
1 cup sugar
1 egg
1 teaspoon bicarbonate soda
1 teaspoon nutmeg (I use a whole nutmeg and grate the quantity needed)
1 teaspoon allspice (I use the whole berries and grind them until I have the right quantity of allspice powder)
pinch of salt

Method

Place the chopped raisins and water in a medium sized saucepan and bring to the boil. Lower heat and add butter. Stir until melted. Turn off the heat and allow the mixture to cool.

When cool, stir the sugar and egg into the raisin mixture in the saucepan. Sift all the dry ingredients and also add to mixture. Mix well to combine, then spread into lamington tray, which has been lined with tin foil and greased. (I use spray oil.)

Bake in a moderate oven (180°C) for approximately 40 minutes.

Cool on rack (if you can wait that long).

Dredge the top of the slice with icing sugar.

In the laundry

Laundry-wise, I had the washing machine and laundry hamper rearranged so that I would be forced to take the dirty washing from the hamper and put it in the machine with my left hand.

For quite a while, Steve hung out and brought in the washing from the clothesline. I began to take the washing off the line when it was dry (as it was also much lighter in weight). This also gave me good practice at raising my arms regularly (and in moderation – I didn't want to go overboard and do damage). I gradually wound the clothesline up fractionally higher each time to increase the height I had to lift my arms.

(Adopting these arm exercises probably sounds ridiculous, but take into consideration that following lymph node removal and mastectomy you are supposed to begin activities again by carrying a set of house/car keys, gradually working up to a handbag!)

Pet therapy

Another arm raising activity was combined with playing with our dog. The puppy we'd bought as a family pet five months before I was diagnosed became a close companion, cuddle-buddy, protector and exercise machine. By the time I'd had my first surgery she had basic obedience skills and was house-trained.

The dog's size and strength increased proportionately to my special needs as I began exercising my right arm more. This was perfect for re-training my arm. I would lie on my back outside on the grass, my arm outstretched, gripping a doggy rope with the dog latched onto the drooly end. She would repeatedly direct my arm up and around to the top of my head in a tug-of-war game, then return back to my side, bringing my arm with her. I would try to pull her in the opposite direction to put some resistance on my arm muscles.

By the time I had my last major surgery, (breast reconstruction, which required a large cut across my abdomen) the 'puppy' was fully grown and particularly excited for me to be home as we'd been apart for a week and a half.

Gaye

Titbit

If you have a 10 kg dog in the home and have been apart due to a recent hospital visit, be careful during the initial re-introduction process especially if you have come straight home from the hospital and gone to bed for a rest. You should be even more careful if a family member opens the back door to let the dog in to see you, but it tears down the hallway into your bedroom before anyone can stop it, leaps up on to the bed – but misses – and actually lands on your stomach, wagging her tail excitedly for you to 'play'. This hurts.

CHAPTER 8

Laughter is the breast medicine

(Chemo and radiotherapy)

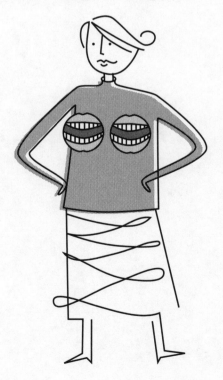

Gaye

I'm not naive enough to believe that simply 'laughing' is a panacea for the pain and trauma of breast cancer, surgery, chemo, radiotherapy and their side effects. Forced or empty laughter (laughing just for the sake of laughing) doesn't appear to be a very fulfilling psychological pastime to me.

When there is an awareness and appreciation of positivity first, laughter can become a healthy, natural and spontaneous by-product. I wasn't laughing at the cancer, I was laughing with it – and putting the paradigm of 'the glass half full rather than half empty' into practice. I stopped looking at what I didn't have and concentrated on what I did have.

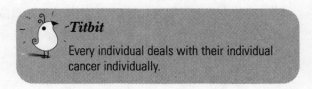

Titbit

Every individual deals with their individual cancer individually.

Because there are so many factors to take into consideration, the fact that you might have the same type of breast cancer, surgery and after-therapy as someone else does not guarantee you will have the same type of experience. That's probably why there is no 'twelve-step program' to follow to get through it. And even if there was, there could never be a guarantee of success or survival for every participant.

In this book alone four very different types of breast cancers are discussed, and they had four different ways of presenting themselves and four different ways of being surgically eliminated.

Just suppose the four women in this book had exactly the same type and class of breast cancer – the same surgery, the same adjuvant therapy. We wouldn't have all had the same outcomes. The fact that we are four different people ensures that we won't encounter the 'same' experience. We are made up of totally different childhood and life experiences, unique to each one of us. These colour and influence the ways in which we behave, see, feel and understand every component in the universe. From the way we relate to others to the mental, physical and spiritual dynamics going on within our own bodies, we will never encounter exactly the same situation.

Since diagnosis, I had primed myself psychologically for the necessary adjuvant (supplementary) therapies, and was prepared to undertake them if it meant removing any trace of cancerous cells.

I came into contact with a number of women after my diagnosis who had had lumpectomies or single mastectomies but who had not been recommended any chemo or radio treatment following their surgery. This disturbed me greatly. I thought, 'I would be *demanding* chemo. I want peace of mind that everything has been done to eradicate every last possible remaining cancer cell.'

After the mastectomy I was referred to an oncologist (a doctor who specialises in tumours and prescribes adjuvant therapy). After examining me and deliberating over my pathology reports, he decided non-recommendation of adjuvant chemotherapy. (That's oncologist talk. Put simply it means 'No chemo.')

He explained that because I had taken the wise step of removing all breast tissue and that the cancer had not moved into the lymph nodes, the possibility of any recurrence in the future would be low – within the region of 12 to 15 per cent. (This was regarded as pretty good. It was approximately the same statistics as that for 'normal' pre-cancer women.) Chemotherapy – if it worked on me – would only decrease that chance by a maximum amount of 3 per cent. Therefore I needed to weigh up that possible 3 per cent benefit with the related possibility of illness and hair loss from the treatment.

I had prepared myself for those side effects so to me that was a non-issue. However, the oncologist also highlighted some information on the long-term effects of chemo, explaining that many drugs used in chemotherapy not only induce early menopause, but are actually able to cause a cancer further on down the track.

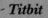

Titbit

Not everyone loses their hair during chemo.
It depends on the cocktail of drugs the
oncologist prescribes for your particular regime.

This information still left me in two minds as to which direction to take. If I wanted chemo he would certainly put the wheels in motion for it to begin, and I would know I had done everything humanly possible to kill off any remaining cancer cells. But I felt I was far too young for the associated problems of menopause, let alone another cancer. Once was enough thanks.

Over the next few days I debated with myself over what to do. Steve was pleased with what the oncologist had said, having gone through a number of radiation therapy regimes to get rid of his cancer. He reckoned he knew what he'd do in my case. 'But Gaye, you've got to do what you feel is right for you … and I'll back you 100 per cent.'

I thought back to my meeting with Sir Galahad after my cancer was diagnosed. His first words were 'What made you have that first mammogram in April 1995?' I told him that while I was at an appointment with Dr Smith we decided it would be wise to check my breasts as well. To Dr Smith, the right breast in particular felt 'nodular' so he insisted I immediately have a mammogram. The results came back with the all clear.

I can remember looking at that mammogram when I got home. I'd immediately noticed a large, prominent, solitary, white 'star-like' effect with long tentacle arms reaching out in a number of different directions. I thought at the time, 'That's a really strange area – and there isn't a matching star in the other breast – but at least the report didn't say it was cancer.'

I relegated the X-ray to my bottom drawer thinking it may come in handy some time in the future. Then Galahad asked to see it following my more recent mammogram.

We asked him why it was relevant. He motioned with his pen towards the big white star on the old X-ray, while Steve and I looked on, and he said, 'See this area here? That's the tumour.'

We stared open-mouthed as he then began pointing to clusters of vivid white 'grains of salt' dotted against the blackness of the X-ray. These were micro-calcifications – pre-cancers. If all these abnormalities were so clearly visible then surely the specialist who checked the mammogram – and holds the responsibility of writing up the results – should have been able to identify them too. (Subsequently, when Dr Smith read out the report findings from the X-ray Centre to me it read '… no pathological calcifications were demonstrated … breast normal'. So, poor old

Smithy had been wrongly informed too. The possible ramifications of anyone, doctor or patient, referring to a report like that for a recommendation on how to treat any future breast problems are frightening.)

I am fully aware that people can and do make mistakes. (I'm inn that catigory myself!) However, if something as obvious as that large tenticled star was overlooked then there is certainly something going on that warrants assessment and correction. I don't put people on pedestals and I don't treat doctors as gods because they're everyday people like you and me. However, I am still at a loss to understand how this 'specialist' (a person who has been trained and consequently has a lot of knowledge in one particular field, as opposed to a general practitioner who has bits of knowledge in lots of fields) had failed to read the signs.

Bewildered, I told Galahad that the pathology report for that earlier mammogram stated I was clear; I had no abnormalities.

To Galahad, it was instantly evident that there were suspicious markings on the X-ray. He said, 'Well, I'm amazed. It's a miracle the tumour has grown so slowly in the amount of time it's been in there.'

When a decision hinges on a report, the information in that report has got to be accurate.

I began to wonder (as opposed to worry) whether the information in the histology reports the oncologist was going by for the basis of his prognosis to chemotherapy was correct. Even though he had been

Gaye

highly recommended to me, I decided I should seek out a second opinion.

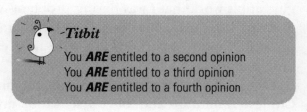

Titbit

You **ARE** entitled to a second opinion
You **ARE** entitled to a third opinion
You **ARE** entitled to a fourth opinion

I sought information about two female oncologists of my choice. It was suggested that one of them would most likely give me chemo no matter what my final choice was. That didn't seem objective enough to me so I went with the other one.

She agreed with the first oncologist we'd seen, citing that my '... prognosis ... could not be substantially improved by adding chemotherapy ...'

After I explained to her my concern about the legitimacy of the actual report she took a further step and arranged to physically examine the histology slides from my frozen section under the microscope to ascertain, for my benefit, the validity of the report. When I phoned a week later and listened to her findings, I felt justified and had peace of mind that non-recommendation of chemotherapy was the correct choice. (Thank you Jacquie.)

Sandy

I went through premature menopause while I was having my chemo and radiotherapy. Jim had told the guys at his work that I was having problems with these dreadful hot flushes and sweating all the time. One of the guys kindly sent me home a peaked cap with a little built-in fan.

One night, twelve of us went out for dinner to a Chinese restaurant and, of course, I took my cap with me. Each time I had a hot flush I would put my cap with the fan on, while everyone at our table turned the event into a 'cool Sandy down' ceremony, and helped by taking up their placemats and fanning me.

Diane

I had six months of chemo that began with a two-week course of tablets. During that fortnight, both times on Monday, I was admitted into hospital (in the evening) to have a drip inserted. They'd run the chemo-cocktail and other assorted drugs through the drip. I stayed overnight for a rest, and the whole process seemed to run quite smoothly.

I found chemotherapy not to be anywhere near as bad as I had imagined it to be. Having said that, I know mine was low grade; it wasn't 'the big whammy'. I did have a number of small side effects, none of which were pleasant, but I managed to keep working part-time; I was able to still help up at the school and I still did my normal motherly things. It's just that I was becoming increasingly tired.

It's probably not really till you're at the end of chemo, when you start to get better, that you realise just how awful you've been feeling or how tired you actually were. They certainly weren't the worst six months of my life. I had expected them to be, but they definitely weren't. Actually the best thing to happen during this six-month period was 'coffee'. Coffee with the girlfriends after dropping the kids off at school in the morning – truly – talking, laughter and great friends were the best medicine.

One of my girlfriends came and sat throughout every chemo session with me while Alan held the fort with the boys at home. As if it wasn't enough just for Debbie to be there, occasionally she'd bring a little something she'd made – a couple of biscuits that she'd baked or a flower picked from her garden. She was terrific; a truly amazing woman.

During my first visit, one of the pre-chemo drugs they gave me was purposely injected into my arm catheter very slowly. Dr Jacquie said, 'Some people find this particular drug gives them a funny tingling sensation in a certain part of their body.'

I asked, 'Are you going to elaborate on that?'

She said, 'No – but if you get it, you'll know.'

So I sat there, waiting, when all of a sudden I became extremely alert.

'Ohhh, ye-e-ss ... Getting it now!'

It's a tingling sensation all around your vaginal and vulval area – like pins and needles. Very sharp ones. And if they push that drug in fast, it's vicious. It hits you like – WHAM!

After that first one, I used to say to Dr Jacquie, 'Just put it in very slowly Jacquie; *ve-ry* slow-ly,' and she'd creep it in. For each of the twelve sessions after that, Debbie would watch me, and right on cue she'd say, 'Mmm. I think it's starting about ... *now*!'

Doris

I didn't have chemotherapy or radiotherapy – either time, incidentally. I don't know why and it never occurred to me to ask. I was just grateful that I didn't have to have it.

Gaye

Most people I've met who have gone through chemo and/or radiotherapy complain that one of the annoying side effects is memory loss.

I had neither therapy, still I admit to having suffered a dreadful loss of memory.

Prior to my cancer I used to be an avid trivia buff. For example, I knew all the words to 'The Patty Duke Show' and knew the names (not just the nicknames) of all the castaways on 'Gilligan's Island' and I *always* knew where I had left my car keys. Now, I forget what I'm talking about mid-sentence and place the stuffed chicken into a roasting dish with about half a cup of water. I've decided to put it all down to a transformational shift in my priorities. My brain, lightly dusted with seasoned flour, doesn't need so much trivia. Inconsequential things are not that important to me now.

CHAPTER 9

Scarved for life

(Hair loss)

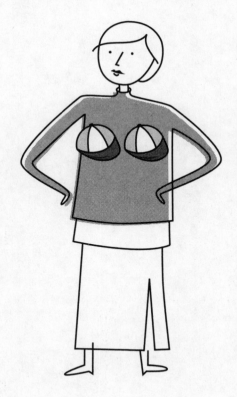

Gaye

My own hair has been described as 'Nicole Kidman' and 'Julia Roberts' (although I call it *my* hair). At the time of diagnosis my hair was the longest it had ever been.

The day Sir Galahad told me about the cancer and chemotherapy, and I cried at the thought of losing my beautiful hair, I became equally determined not to become a stereotypical turbaned advertisement for the disease. If I had to lose my Kidman-esque hair, I would do it with a style of my choosing.

I'd look like one of the characters in *Romper Stomper*, complete with shaved head, black boots, ripped jeans and white tee-shirt. I even went out and bought a couple of faux nose and eyebrow rings!

Ordinarily I wouldn't go out of my way to shave my head to make a statement of individuality. But now, confronted with a situation that enabled me to see just how precious, profound and fleeting life is, I had the opportunity to make decisions based on a glorious combination of nouveau bravado, joy of life and an abandonment of consequences. I had the courage to feel good about finally getting rid of accumulated and hoarded possessions – not to be confused with a 'preparing for death' cleanout. I also experienced a sense of mischievous invincibility – not a 'tempting fate' scenario, more like, 'Hey! I've got cancer. What can anyone do to me?' It gave me an excuse to run through shopping centres and pinch strangers' bottoms.

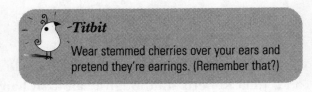

Titbit

Wear stemmed cherries over your ears and pretend they're earrings. (Remember that?)

Soon after the lumpectomy I made an appointment to see my hairdresser to make sure I had a decently shaped head for baldness. She felt all over my scalp, pulled my hair back at different angles and gave a resounding 'Yes'.

Chemo-chic! We arranged that I would return a few weeks before chemo began for a short-cropped rogue helipad hairstyle. This way, not only would baldness be an easier transition (for me and those around me – particularly the kids), but it would also prevent the continual vacuuming up of my long strands of hair falling out in dribs and drabs all over the carpet.

Initially it was an anti-climax when the oncologist gave the recommendation of 'no chemotherapy' because I was at the stage where I felt totally comfortable with the prospect of baldness, and now I wouldn't be able to go through with all my preparations of nose rings, hairstyles (or lack of) and scalp pictures. I had even taken Elissa and Kerrie to our local butcher shop and pointed to one of the butchers, showing the type of hairstyle I planned to get prior to baldness. Fortunately the kids approved of the radical style and thought I'd look pretty cool – especially when I came up to the school to help with reading.

Oh well, no chemo was a bonus, so I shouldn't grumble. And if I really had wanted to go bald voluntarily there was always a seat at the hairdresser's with my name on it. (I'd better see about getting that removed.)

Sandy

The oncologist said to me, 'Go and get your wig before we start chemotherapy.' So I bought my wig, but it's something I don't think anybody wants to do on their own. Sharon came with me and we sat outside the hair studio for a little while before we went in. (I must confess we were a bit teary.) I thought, 'This is it. I'm going to buy a wig.' Then I got all uppity and said, 'Well I'm going to buy the best and the most expensive wig; it's going to cost me thousands of dollars for this real-hair-wig.'

When I got in there and relaxed a little, I thought, 'Oh, this is bloody ridiculous. I'm only going to wear it for a few months' (because your hair grows back really quickly).

The girls at the hair studio couldn't have been more helpful. They took me into a cubicle and I must have tried on about 20 or 30 wigs. At one stage I even decided I was going to go red! I've always wanted to be a redhead. I thought, 'If I'm going to lose my hair, I'm going to make a real statement about it.'

In the end though, I actually bought a wig similar in length and colour to my own hair. I couldn't bring it home till it was ready because they were going to cut and style it to make it look natural.

When I finally got it home I thought, 'Oh dear, I don't know about this.' It had a bit more grey in it where my hair was more blonde, and I didn't know that I truly liked it. So I rang the studio the next day and explained my doubts to them.

'Oh, that's all right,' they said. 'Bring it back and we'll try something else.' They were absolutely fantastic.

So off I tootled and had my first hit of chemo. About two weeks later, when I was sitting up in bed having my morning coffee, I ran my fingers through my hair. I pulled my hand back suddenly and all this hair was hanging from my fingers. I said to myself, 'Oh my goodness; this is it.' Then I thought, 'Okay, fine; that's all right.'

I had already spoken to my hairdresser and she was wonderful. She said, 'As soon as you feel you want to come in, we'll go out to the back room.' (The oncologist had suggested I have my hair cut right back to my scalp, without shaving it, to avoid my hair constantly dropping onto the floor.) Along I went to the salon wearing my wig. I said to my hairdresser, 'Today's the day!'

'Okay,' she said, 'out we go.' She was in a worse state than I was. She was trying not to cry, and we're laughing and trying to think of all these stupid things to say while she's going *zzzzzzzz* over the top of my head.

And all my beautiful hair – I felt like picking it up and sticking it all back on again. But it was much better with it off. I put my wig back on and walked out of the shop again. And she didn't charge me for that haircut, bless her heart.

The night that I had my hair cut off, I put my wig back on when Jim came home from work.

I was lying on the couch near the glass doors and waved to him as he came through the gate. He was carrying so many things in his arms at the time that he

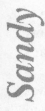*Sandy*

wasn't able to wave back. He got to the door and bent down to put a carton of milk on the ground so that he could open the door. While his head was down I whipped my wig off!

Then he stood up. Well, I just about gave him a stroke.

One minute I've got a head full of hair and the next, I look like a plucked chicken!

The only hair that didn't fall out was the hair on my legs! You'd think they'd get the message after nearly 40 years of shaving, wouldn't you? They refused to die!

I decided that if I was going to go through all this, I had to look absolutely stunning!

I went back to the hair studio and bought some lovely turbans. The girls there also showed me how to do beaut things with scarves.

Then I popped along to a market and bought some earrings like you couldn't imagine. They were the most hideous big things that hung from my earlobe right down to my shoulder. Jim swore, vowed and declared that if ever I walked out the door with them on, he'd never ever talk to me again.

They were the most appalling earrings I could find, and I did wear them a few times, I don't mind telling you. I probably went a bit overboard with those. They were utterly grotesque but they were only two dollars

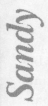

each – I suppose they'll be fun for the grandchildren to dress up in one day.

I think somebody else must have had chemo and when all their hair dropped out they decided they desperately needed earrings, so went into business!

My youngest son, Craig, was going out with this lass who had a Ford Capri with a fold-down roof.

He brought this magnificent new car around to our place and said to Jim, 'Take Mum for a drive in it.' A beautiful day it was, so we jumped in the car, put down the roof and off we drove to visit some friends a couple of streets away. They're absolute car freaks so they thought this car was really great stuff.

When we were saying goodbye, Jim backed the car out the driveway and as he took off at a great speed, I whipped off my wig!

We're blazing down the straight and there I am totally bald and waving my hair around in the air over my head!

Well they nearly died. To this day, they still keep telling the story of Sandy with her wig off!

I think you have to make the most of it, because you'd go crazy otherwise.

Diane

I lost half my hair. I don't mean I lost great big handfuls; it just thinned out to half my hair volume. The texture changed somewhat but I still had hair. Enough not to have to worry about turbans and scarves, so that was very comforting because from what I've seen, most women find that a really difficult issue. It's not so much that you've lost the hair for yourself; it's that you become instantly recognisable as a cancer patient – just a further blow to an already vulnerable self-image.

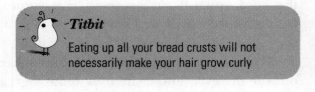

Titbit

Eating up all your bread crusts will not necessarily make your hair grow curly

CHAPTER 10

My cups runneth over

(Prostheses)

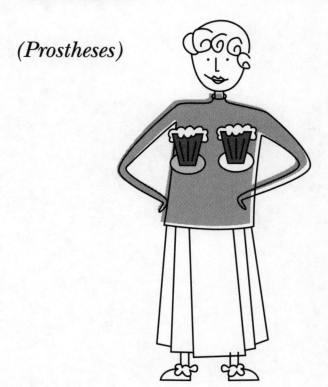

Gaye

Someone suggested I wear a 'little padded bra, so that my flat chest wouldn't make other people feel uncomfortable.'

Other people? ... Uncomfortable?!

Stuff *that* hadegaloony!

This thing happened to me and I was dealing with it. When I looked down at my chest I felt perfectly comfortable. If other people couldn't cope with it – if they have to worry about the size of my breasts, then they're the ones with the problem.

And I didn't think a handful of stuffing was going to fix it.

Long before the mastectomy I had decided I wasn't going to bother with padding.

Even at that early stage, I had no problem with the thought of being flat, let alone the reality. And after the event I think I even surprised myself at my acceptance of being flat-chested. I loved being flat. For me, it was a totally liberating experience.

I felt as if I was taller. I *was* taller. I walked taller. Gone was the extra mass being pulled down by gravitational forces. (I 'lost' around four kilograms in one afternoon!) Over 15 years' worth of daily head-aches disappeared. I no longer knocked myself unconscious when I danced or drove over speed humps. It was bliss being able to lie comfortably on my stomach. Going from a five-hook bra to no bra at all was just the best.

There was absolutely no trauma, embarrassment or shame associated with the whole thing for me whatsoever, nor did I have any feelings of being 'disfigured'. There were so many advantages I couldn't see any disadvantages. I didn't worry about what I *didn't* have because I was too busy being thankful for what I *did* have. My glass was always half full and my (bra) cups were full and running over.

A nurse told me of a mastectomy lady she knew who made her own prostheses by filling small nylon pantyhose bags with bird seed and fastening them inside her bra-cups. (The weight of the seeds offered a natural bosomy weight and drape.)

Apparently, this lady wore her seed prostheses under her bathers while she went swimming and the subsequent humid weather caused them to sprout!

She was last seen being chased by a pack of vegetarians.

Sandy

We're talking nearly 20 years ago since my mum had her mastectomy. Mum was reasonably well endowed but too proud to go to the mastectomy clinic to get a decent prosthesis. Being a dressmaker, she decided to make her own. She lined the inside of her empty bra-cup and padded it out with cotton wool.

Well, my son Craig, who was a little boy at the time, discovered that he could sit on grandma's knee and manoeuvre this boob thing around. He'd always be touching her. He'd push it here; it would shoot up there and move around to here. Craig really took a shine to that boob; he thought it was great!

Diane

I tried the 'stick-on' prosthesis but after a while I discovered I had a skin allergy to the 'sticky' part. Also, because I was fairly large breasted I needed a large prosthesis to match. I noticed the extreme weightiness of it which pulled down on the skin of my chest, unlike a real breast where you wouldn't be aware of the weight being so uncomfortable.

Diane

And I wasn't ever really happy with my 'pop-down-the-top' prosthesis. I felt it moved around too much. I was constantly aware of it wandering about inside my bra.

It sapped my confidence because I was forever having to make sure the prosthesis was in its proper place. If I even bent slightly forward it would move from its original position so I was forever putting my hand down the front of my top to adjust it.

On one occasion I was planting seedlings in a garden bed in the front yard near to where my oldest son was shooting hoops with a basketball. I'd watered the soil and dug in some mulch and manure through the dirt. I had my rubber gloves on and I was right into it.

Everything was going well until I ever so slightly changed the way I was moving or bending (without remembering to make allowances for the fact that my prosthesis enjoyed dancing up a storm inside my bra cup). The next minute I heard a dull splat. I looked down to see my prosthesis laying in the garden bed gazing back up at me. (It had made its way up over the top of my bra, down inside my tee-shirt, and fallen into the mucky dirt.)

As I stared at my prosthesis, my instant thought was, 'I want to die.'

I felt so exposed – so vulnerable. I wanted to cry, but my next thought was, 'I'm stuck here in the front yard … and there are people around.' Immediately I was conscious that if I stood up to walk back to the house to escape, anybody passing by would be perfectly aware that I had a huge single breast.

Not a good look!

(Actually, looking back, no one would have noticed anything – it was just how insecure I was feeling.)

I looked at my muddy gloves and I thought, 'I can't even pick up the prosthesis and carry it inside.'

I called my son, Craig, over and asked if he could help me for a second. He said, 'Sure Mum, what's the problem?'

I told him, 'My prosthesis has fallen out …'

He walked over to the grubby boob, which was still sitting in the mud. 'That's all right; don't worry about it,' he said. 'I'll get it for you.'

And he picked up the prosthesis from the mud, carefully cradling it as he carried it (with me following close behind) all the way to the house. I awkwardly snapped off the dirty gloves and dumped them at the doorstep, slipping in through the front door so that I could quickly take my prosthesis to the nearest tap.

As I washed it I thought, 'That's it!' Because while I could see the funny side of the situation and laugh at it I was also aware of the sensitivity and the caring that my son had shown me.

It dawned on me that the same thing could very easily happen again. It could pop out at the school or the shops – anywhere! And that would be the end of me; it would destroy me. It was beginning to affect my confidence level. So that was the first crunch.

Diane

Before two weeks had passed I was hanging clothes out on the washing line and the bugger fell out again! At least this time it landed in the washing basket and stayed clean and relatively dry. But it made me realise that it could happen somewhere unexpectedly, and it would not be a comfortable situation.

For me, the decision to get a breast reconstruction was not so much a physical requirement as a practical one. Surgery would alleviate the problems I had with my prosthesis making travel arrangements without bothering to consult me first, which would therefore solve the associated confidence issues.

Doris

After the removal of the first breast I spent a great deal of time learning to balance the real me with the plastic me. Balance is a problem you see, because the shoulder on the weight-free no-bosom side tends to stand up much higher than the heavy bosomy side.

Doris

When I first began looking for a false boob I read the literature and it said something about, 'Some women may get a handkerchief and sew pebbles into it …' (a handkerchief mind, not 'a bit of fabric' but a handkerchief!)

So I tried that, and popped it into my bra. I ended up with small blisters and terrible chafing on the skin of my chest, so I abandoned that idea.

Another prosthesis I'd heard about was made of birdseed – but I had the sudden image of being in a movie, pursued by thousands of birds trying to peck at me, so I gave up on that idea too.

Then I found an Australian invention; a piece of sheepskin – the wool went against your chest, and the rounded booby side was covered with silky knicker fabric. It was filled with little stones. The idea behind the stones was to give you the weight of a breast. So I bought one of those, tucked it into my bra, and two things happened.

The first thing I discovered happened while I was engrossed in conversation with somebody one day. Every time I turned my face to the right, my nose began to itch. It took a while to realise that the wool bosom had wriggled out of my bra, and I had half a sheep poking up my nostril.

The second discovery occurred when I went to visit a friend. This lady was extremely house proud and she'd recently had the flooring replaced and varnished in the hallway, along with a number of other rooms of the house. Beautiful jarrah floorboards.

They were absolutely stunning. She also had exquisite furniture in the rooms and wonderful expensive light fittings.

She met me at the front door and stood back to let me in – but before I could venture a step forward, this huge golden retriever bounded up from behind me and made his way in through the door.

The woman frantically began waving her arms about, pleading, 'Don't let him in, don't let him in!' But it was too late. The dog was inside, and the woman conceded defeat with, 'Oh well, I don't suppose it matters. It's just that he lives around the back of the house, where we've only got old carpet.' (Old carpet, indeed!)

Then she led me across her magnificent hallway. She just wanted to show off her new flooring, and I was very happy to look at it. We hadn't walked very far on the grand tour when in between the commentary I became aware of these peculiar little crunching noises. Finally we arrived at the kitchen and I suddenly realised what the noise was.

The gravel in my false breast had cut its way through the fabric, and sprinkled to the floor – and as I walked from room to room I had been unwittingly crunching and grinding the little stones into the first seven layers of floor polish.

The woman stopped talking and looked back in absolute horror at this trail of pulverised muck on her beautiful new floorboards and gasped 'Oh no, what's that?'

I looked about the floor and offered helpfully, 'Goodness. I wonder if it was the dog!'

After that I decided to try a wooden breast. I know a man who works with wood. (He makes bowls and things out of those knobbly bits on trees.) I drew the kind of size I wanted and asked him whether he could make it.

'Probably,' he said. 'What do you want it for?'

I answered, 'A breast.'

In the end he persuaded me that it was a silly idea. But three months later he sent me one. It was a very small boob but it had a two-inch-long nipple sticking out from the middle of it. I mean it stuck so far out, you could have hung anything on it – three Christmas hams and a dressing gown! So that wasn't such a good idea.

I finally settled on a very pert little French set. Terribly expensive, and they even had the suggestion of a nipple moulded into them. They're full of a jelly of some sort (lime flavour I suspect) and the idea was that when you lie down the prosthesis breast also flattens out slightly. Mind you, when I did lie down, my own breast (which was about four sizes larger than the jellied variety) was still standing up at attention! That was all very well until one day I went to the beach and the jelly boob floated out of my bathing costume.

Doris

I got a brand new pair of prostheses when I was 59, after my second lump was diagnosed as cancer and that breast came off as well. I was also left with lymphoedema so I've had to wear an elasticised compression 'sleeve' ever since – to help control the swelling in my left arm.

> ### Titbit
>
> Fill out and wear a medical talisman in the event of unconsciousness or an accident. It is imperative that you are not administered an injection or blood pressure reading from the arm which has had the lymph glands removed or you could end up with lymphoedema.
>
> There is no cure for lymphoedema: only prevention.

The elastic strap (which holds the sleeve up) passes across my chest, nestles just under my right armpit, across my back and finally attaches to the back of the 'sleeve'.

Initially the only problem with it was that because I no longer had my own breasts, there weren't any natural deterrents to stop the chest strap from slowly riding upward and pushing everything out of its way. So the prostheses would gently slither out from the bra cups and out over the top of my bra.

Laughing made the problem even worse. I found that the vibrations of laughter compelled the chest strap to slide upward even faster, causing the prostheses to abruptly 'pop out' of my bra.

One time, in particular, I was out at a restaurant with a group of girlfriends for lunch – and I was having Caesar salad. (I remember that perfectly well, because salad is a rarity for me; I usually order chips.) We were all talking and falling about with laughter when all of a sudden one of my boobs popped out, coming to rest on top of my Caesar salad.

Well I knew exactly what it was and what had happened but the other women didn't. One of them looked over at my plate and asked, 'Did you order that?'

Another woman stared at my plate and scoffed, '*That's* not chicken breast!'

'No, it's not *chicken* breast,' I said, lifting it from the lettuce, 'it's *Doris* breast.'

That was the day I decided I might as well not bother any more with breasts and bras.

A lady told me about her prosthesis incident. She was in her early 30s and she'd had a breast removed. One day while she was doing the housework she saw the young minister from church arrive at the front gate. She asked her four-year-old daughter, Emily, to open the front door for Mr So-and-so while she hurried upstairs to the bedroom to put on her bra, bosom and a clean tee-shirt. She searched frantically for the boob, while Emily let the minister in and sweetly explained, 'Mummy's tumming.'

After some time, being unable to find it she gave up the hunt and put a cardigan on to cover the empty space on her chest. She wandered back downstairs to the living room, where Emily and the minister were sitting on the sofa – and there was the false boob! It was in the minister's hand, and he was drawing a face on it with texta-colour.

Now why he would think that any mother would give her child a limbless, bodiless and faceless Cabbage Patch doll, I can't imagine!

Another woman told me she'd spent months looking for her prosthesis, only to eventually discover that the dog had buried it. The dog had never taken to burying things before so the woman thought that she must have lost it or accidentally thrown it out. Finally her husband found the boob – coming up through the soil among the daffodils.

CHAPTER 11

Making mountains out of molehills

(Breast reconstruction)

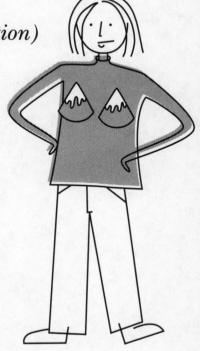

Gaye

Transverse Rectus Abdominus Myocutaneous Flap, otherwise known as a TRAM Flap, is a method of breast reconstruction that uses the patient's own tissue (taking the skin, fat and blood vessels from the tummy area) to create a new breast after mastectomy.

Briefly, it involves removing the tummy tuck material from the abdomen, along with a portion of fat, muscle and the blood vessels. This jigsaw of flesh is known as a 'flap' and is transferred to the breast site. The blood vessels of the flap are connected to an artery vein from the chest wall using microsurgery, which allows the blood supply to recirculate inside the 'new breast'. A synthetic mesh graft is incorporated into the tummy region to strengthen the abdominal wall. A new umbilicus (belly button) is formed and the abdomen is closed.

> There was a young redhead named Gaye;
> They cut half her tummy away.
> They grabbed two big bits,
> And made brand new tits
> And now they don't sag, swing, or sway!
> (Linda Haggar)

I did not have a breast reconstruction to raise my self-esteem, to make me a 'whole' person, or to please my husband. Both of us were thoroughly comfortable with my chest the way it was. The mastectomy and everything that surrounded the experience was never traumatic for me. I felt, and still feel, no psychological anguish. This was probably because we never looked at it in terms of losing a breast. We saw it as saving me.

I found so many advantages to being super flat and I was extremely proud of my mastectomy scars. (Steve said that they were my 'beauty-marks'.) And the scars didn't remind me of having no breasts, or of being disfigured in any way; instead they told me, 'You have done this to extend your life. Well done!'

My motive for reconstruction was primarily to get rid of my now obvious wobbly belly – the boobs were pudding!

I had no intention of using artificial substances inside me to form new bosoms so, from the remnants of two pregnancies without post-birth sit-ups, I was able to supply my chest with the necessary materials from my tummy (seeing there were a couple of spare metres on each roll). I knew I would never get my belly back to a desirable shape through dieting and exercise. I had tried in the past, but there was always that extra bit left that just wouldn't budge.

After I'd announced I was definitely going ahead with the breast reconstruction I was amazed at how many ladies on the spur of the moment said, 'You'll feel just like a woman again!'

How horrible! It made me aware that I had never

even considered myself as not feeling like or *being* a woman. Maybe they live by the breastistentialist philosophy of, 'I have breasts, therefore I am.'

Am I the one who's missing something here (besides lactation ducts)? What is it that causes people to think that a woman is no longer a woman just because a breast or two is missing?

I met a young woman who was due to have a hysterectomy to remove uterine cancer. She sadly, and inaccurately, depicted herself as a hermaphrodite – no longer woman but not quite a man.

I'm glad I don't have the unrealistic view that femininity and womanhood are intrinsically linked to breasts. Having my outer accessories removed didn't make me feel any less a woman or a sexual being. My husband certainly didn't see me as any less desirable, physically or sensually, due to my lack of rack. The mastectomy only took away my flesh, not my femaleness.

Oddly enough, I found that men had a better accepting attitude about the whole boob removal thing than women. (Even though many men can't actually pronounce the word 'breast', they told me, 'If my wife/woman had what you had, I'd want her to do what you did.') The general reaction from men seemed to be, 'Oh, wow!' From women (as they clutched at their own twin-set), it was, 'Oh, no!'

Some of the blokes at Steve's work made me a wonderful catalogue displaying a variety of breasts from magazines, to take with me when I saw the plastic surgeon. There was the 'Super Model' range, the

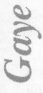

'Pamela Lee' range, and my favourite – the 'Sara Lee' range. (Mmm ... cheesecake!)

Steve was able to accompany me to see each of the reconstructive plastic surgeons on my shopping list.

The first surgeon was terrific. He explained everything honestly, right down to the rarely mentioned failure statistics. 'The percentage of cases that don't work out due to surgical complications or rejection (by your own body) is 10 per cent. But you need to realise Gaye, that if the operation is not a success for you, that is a 100 per cent failure rate for you personally.'

He also had the most gorgeous pair of small hands. 'Beautiful equipment for such a delicate procedure,' I thought. But his 10 to 12-hour time-frame for the operation was extremely daunting. (Not only did I feel that this was a terribly long time to be under anaesthetic, I couldn't help wondering how many trips to the bathroom he would need during such a lengthy amount of time.)

I got the impression from surgeon number two that he didn't appreciate my husband being with me. Apart from virtually ignoring Steve, I felt the doctor's questions seemed a tad stupid. He read my referral, which stated that I'd had a mastectomy, and was now contemplating reconstructive surgery. He looked at me with the depth of a B-grade American talk-show-host-cum-psychologist and said, 'You've lost both breasts, Gaye. (Pause, turn head, mid-shot to camera four.) How does that make you feel?'

I restrained myself from the sarcasm of replying 'Well *duh*! Apart from *preserving my life*, I've had to sell my collection of silk nipple tassels and sequined pasties.'

He was reputed to be a wonderful surgeon, but I knew he wasn't for me.

I put my breasts-to-be in the hands of the third surgeon, Mr 'call me Geoff'. Both Steve and I liked him. He was normal; a modest, down-to-earth human being, who spoke to us without condescension or medical palaver. There was no need to look any further.

He shook Steve's hand vigorously and said, 'It's terrific to see the husband included in something like this.' I felt that if he could support my husband, how much greater would his support be for me, his patient.

As with the first surgeon, we were shown an array of slides (showing the before and after views of surgery, as well as a small number of failures). There was a lengthy explanation of the procedure, followed the mandatory examination of my belly for the surgeon to see what he would be working with.

'Oh yes!' he said enthusiastically, 'This'll be a piece of cake!'

He preferred to work with a partner, which would drastically slash operating time down to between five and six hours. This seemed to me to be a much better time frame.

Talking about the preferred size of the finished product, I told him that there was no way I wanted to be as large as I had been originally. I had in mind a perky set in a C cup. He stepped backwards and looked again at the volume of donor material, scratched his chin, then said earnestly, 'I reckon we can get a pair of Ds with that.'

I wasn't sure whether to be flattered, or to dust off my ab-worker.

Because Mr Geoff has the highest intentions for his surgical result to be aesthetically pleasing, as well as successful, he sent me off to see a number of medicos who would be involved during and after surgery. I booked in for a variety of chest X-rays and ultrasounds to make sure the delicate vessels, which would be joined up to transport blood flow to my new bosoms, would be a useable size. (The problem of vessels shrinking after a mastectomy causes lengthy undue interruptions during the reconstruction. This surgeon wanted to be prepared before surgery for every contingency, and both Steve and I appreciated that.)

It was also important to begin collecting blood. Autologus (my own) blood was collected and stored in the likely event it would be required during the operation and for post-surgery transfusion. Using my own blood eliminated the risk of rejection, which would be an unnecessary ordeal in an already physically traumatic situation.

During the month before reconstruction it was imperative to start special breathing exercises under the guidance of a physiotherapist. This was probably even more critical than the reserve of blood supplies and the necessity of the X-rays put together.

Jack, the physio I was referred to, explained the importance and consequences of the exercises – which were to be practised daily for a month before surgery, then put into effect immediately after I regained consciousness. The breathing exercises would train my lungs to expand to their full capacity. After surgery, it would be natural for me to take short, shallow breaths, but this was exactly what had to be avoided. Shallow breathing uses only the top section of the lungs. Without oxygen being fully deployed, the basal (lower) sections begin to close down and the lungs collapse on themselves. Therefore the condition of my lungs was scrutinised constantly after surgery, and the barrage of encouragement to 'breathe deeper' came from all directions.

My expectations of breezing through the reconstruction by continuing to look for the positives and have a good laugh almost failed. (It's probably fair to say that after the operation I felt as if I'd been hit by a TRAM – a number 86 city-bound tram.)

From day one to day five after the operation, in between experiencing blurs of day and night, my body was wracked with inescapable pain. This was interspersed with bouts of teary depression, involuntary spasms caused by narcotics, and the annoying necessity of 12 feeding and drainage tubes going to and from various bags and bottles.

Combined with the urgent cries from staff to, 'breathe, Gaye, breathe,' I wondered when I would ever laugh again. Occasionally I felt small twinges of positiveness but they became trapped in the vortex of pain – and drowned. (It took me six weeks before I started thinking that the operation and pain were worth the result of a flat tummy and having boobs again. And as time goes on, I am glad that I went through with it.)

I drifted in and out of sleep during the initial days after surgery, but I was conscious of the dedication and compassion of one nurse who spent time sitting beside my bed just holding my hand. I can't recall what he said at the time or whether he said anything at all, but I remember that simple act being the most comforting experience during those nine days in hospital. (Thank you, Lindsay.)

The nurses and physio-terrorists took turns with a specialised breathing machine during the days and nights after the operation, which forced my breathing to use more lung capacity than I was occupying through my own abilities.

'Come on, Gaye,' Jack the physio would urge, 'we have to breathe deeper ... hold that breath ... 2 ... 3 ... 4 ... Slow-ly release. Fantastic. We're doing *really* well!'

'We?' I thought. Well I don't know about me, but he didn't seem to be suffering too much from having had his chest and belly ripped open!

I couldn't be consoled by Jack's bubbling enthusiasm; it hurt too much.

'How's our breathing going?' Jack would ask every time he passed by my room. Then before I could answer, he'd bring his dimples and stethoscope into the room and listen to my lungs, just to make sure I was behaving. 'Great. Get that air right down. We have to expand those basals ...'

Friday night, watching television, I discovered I was finally able to laugh again. That was painful. A nurse wandered in to my room, after hearing the eruptions of laughter followed by the desperate groans of pain. I tried to explain the joke to her, but this hurt even more. She advised me to turn off the television and gave me some tablets for the pain.

I began listening to the radio, thinking it would be a safer alternative. The broadcasters had me in even more stitches than I was already being held together with, so I had to turn that off as well. These incidents (although excruciating) were the cornerstone I desperately needed, to lift my head out of the gloom and walk with my face towards the sunshine.

By Saturday I was finally beginning to feel human again. After lunch Jack stood in the doorway with his broad smile. 'How's our exercise going? I'll just get you to sit up so we can have a listen,' he added, striding into the room adjusting his stethoscope.

By now I was well trained in the procedure, so I slowly manoeuvred myself to sit on the edge of the bed with my back towards him so that he could listen to my lungs. 'That's great; we're doing really well …'

He continued talking as he removed the stethoscope, hung it back around his neck, and walked around the foot of the bed to face me while finishing his dialogue: '… So that's terrific! Now, we'll just get back into bed and …'

'I'll just get back into bed by myself, if you don't mind!' I interrupted, and covered myself up with the sheet. He was momentarily stricken with silence, but slowly through his embarrassed facial expressions I could see that he was slowly becoming aware of what he said. Profuse apologies tumbled out of his mouth along with resolutions to practise saying 'you' rather than 'we' or 'our'.

My last full day in hospital was a memorable one. It was one of those 'they always happen in threes' experiences.

It was the first Tuesday in November – Melbourne Cup Day. (It was also the first time Steve and the girls were actually able to be with me in my room because each of them came down with flu the day after my surgery. Until now, visits had been conducted with me in my room and my family shouting to me from their position outside the fire exit door.) We had a picnic on the bed and each chose horses for the Cup. I'd already been allocated two horses in the Hospital Sweepstakes that morning: 'Might and Power' and another horse ridden by some Italian jockey.

We watched the race on television and I won the first prize payout – twelve dollars and fifty cents!

Then, later after dinner that night, I thought I could smell something burning – something *electrical* burning. I ambled down the corridor to the left of my room, sniffing the air. Nothing. I returned and walked slowly down the corridor to my right, but again nothing.

Thinking I must be going mad, I went back to my room.

'Aaahh … It's in *here*!' The smell was intense and coming from my room. I hobbled as fast as I could to the nurses' office with my 'hip-to-hip' abdominal wound, and asked a group of six nurses whether any of them would mind coming down to have a smell of my room. Two nurses hesitated. (I later found out that they thought I was joking – after all, Tuesday was chicken curry night!)

Four nurses followed me back down to room 14 and began sniffing. After exhausting all possible places in the room where the smell could have originated from they decided to call in the Fire Brigade. I grabbed my most valuable possessions from the room – a photograph of Steve and the girls, and my first prize Cup money – and hurried down to the reception area (nice and handy, next to the front door), just in case evacuation became necessary. I had front row seats to watch the arrival of two massive fire trucks with their lights flashing and sirens wailing.

The staff thought it was certainly one way of celebrating my Cup win – C cup, that is!

One and a half hours after all the firemen started buzzing around with their thermo-vision – heat-seeking toys – the all clear was given. The explanation was something to do with the heating system in the ceiling above my room. (The smell had wafted through the ceiling vent.)

As I made my way back to my room and passed a group of firemen talking with a nurse, I smiled and said, 'Goodnight.' One of the firemen addressed the nurse saying, 'Gee she looks all right; she doesn't even need to be in here.' I smiled and thought to myself, 'If only you knew.'

My third experience of that day happened much, much later that night, when I phoned through to the radio program that had kept me company, to tell the two male broadcasters how sore they had made me on Friday night, and that now I had something in common with them. I explained briefly that I was in hospital having breast reconstructive surgery, following cancer. (They interrupted, vehemently denying that they'd had any breast surgery.)

'So now I've *got* two boobs,' I said, 'and you *are* two boobs!'

They sent me off to a dinner for two at a wonderful seafood restaurant!

Both my breasts went along.

During the fortnight after returning home, nurses came to the house to inspect the wounds and change the dressings. With each new nurse, the moment of viewing my unbandaged bosoms resulted in an instant proclamation of, 'That's a Geoff!'

It was spoken with the same certainty a couture bon vivant might use when proclaiming that a gown is unmistakably Lacroix from among its rivals. (So my new breasts were distinguishable by the hands that shaped them. That made me even prouder, if that was possible.)

I had forgotten to send a birthday card to a very dear aunt of mine while I was in hospital having the reconstruction. I remembered two months later and sent a card expressing belated birthday wishes and my apologies, with a short explanation. 'I had a couple of things on my chest at the time.'

Early December I sent out our Christmas cards with a letter. Here are some excerpts:

Gaye

Monday 8.12.97

Dear Loved One …

… It has been six weeks to the day of the operation, and it's only now that I'm starting to think I made the right choice to go ahead with the reconstruction. The six-hour-long procedure involved using my tummy flab to make two new boobies, and inserting a mesh lining to strengthen the wall of my abdomen. My tummy is nearly back to pre-pregnant flat (still a bit of post-operational swelling), and I have gained the most *fabulous* set of pert bosoms. It's an amazing procedure – taking bits off here, sewing them in there, no stretching or puckering in the seams. Wonderful stuff!

Next step will be the forming of the nipples. Please excuse my bold openness. I reckon I could talk the leg off a chair about the whole episode – but only, I think, because it has been such a positive experience!

Back to the … ahem, nipples …

I will be returning to Geoff who, with the magic of plastic surgery, will perform the procedure, followed by a nurse who 'colours' in the nipple and surrounding areola by tattoo. His name is 'Mad Dog' O'Reilly. Gotcha again. [It's all done by Maxine, a qualified nurse, but that didn't sound exciting enough.]

… Steve, Elissa and Kerrie have been terrific all the way through. We have made sure we have kept our sense of humour, and the girls always want to be informed of what's happening to me. It eases any worries they have and keeps them feeling included.

Steve has been *absolutely* wonderful. I love him *so*

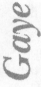Gaye

much. He has been a tower of strength to me and has fully supported all my choices.

Someone at church yesterday asked me whether I still had any pain. I told this bloke, 'The only pain I have is when Steve constantly reminds me how terrifically efficient he is at the housework (because I'm not) and organising the kids for school – before he goes off to work!'

Breast Wishes, Gaye.

One of our friends told us how she'd been sitting at the kitchen table 'laughing her head off' while reading the Christmas letter. Her husband came into the house from the backyard to find out what was so funny. Wiping her eyes, and between broken laughter, she held up the letter and said, 'Gaye's got cancer!'

Six months after the breast reconstruction I returned for the nipple construction.

After I was wheeled down to theatre, the nurse who assisted Mr Geoff as he measured me up (to position the new nipples), called over a number of theatre nurses to come see my 'new breasts'. I showed them off proudly as the group of nurses surrounded the end

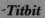
and sides of the bed, staring in awe and cooing like a brood of relatives around a new baby. The comments were practically the same: 'Aren't they *lovely*!' 'Oh Gaye, you *have* done well!' 'Ohh, they're *be-autiful*!' 'The left one definitely takes after its father – have you decided on any names yet?'

The actual nipple construction operation was to take about five minutes (and at the same time, a lumpy piece of necrosis (dead fat), about the size of my thumb, would be removed from the top area of my breast).

The skin on the breast at the pre-approved nipple site would be cut in a specific pattern and manipulated to resemble a (tiny) top hat, then stitched in place. The construction of the areola was a circle of cobweb-looking incisions which, after some time, would provide the dimpled texture surrounding the nipples.

I woke to discover foam doughnuts on top of each breast around the new nipples.

A lollypop stick had been passed through a loosely stitched loop through each nipple (to prevent it from collapsing) and lay across the top of the foam doughnut.

Contrary to the standard wound-care routine, I wasn't to be overly concerned about keeping the new nipples covered and dry while showering, etc. It was more important to 'cure' them – not 'heal' them. This helped to produce a more realistic areola texture and appearance.

When Steve saw them for the first time, he thought they looked like 'a piece of ham after the string netting has been removed'.

I returned almost a year later for the surgeon's nurse to colour in the nipples and areola by tattoo procedure.

I had a pretty good idea of what I wanted: 'GEOFF WAS HERE' (my reconstructive plastic surgeon) in a circle around my right nipple, and 'GAYE LOVES STEVIE XX' around the left nipple, which sits over my heart. (And although many patients would like to have a reminder of Mr Geoff upon their nipple, I was eventually talked into having a 'standard round'.)

Maxine, the nurse, began by showing me her tattoo-ink colour charts. For my skin colour she recommended 'Mac Mauve' for the areola, and 'Dark Pink' for the actual nipple. She explained that the two different shades would make the nipple appear more natural, and offer enhanced visual protrusion to the nipple itself. And aren't protruding nipples on the top of every woman's 'To Do' list?

So. What comes in at number two on the list then?

Having a television crew come along to film it as part of a segment on 'Good Medicine' of course!

I thought the tattooing could be a good opportunity to promote breast cancer awareness. Seeing as I had very little feeling in these new bosoms, and the nipple region appeared so physically authentic, I thought how wincing it would look for such a sensitive area of a woman's body to be bombarded with buzzing tattoo needles. And if there were any women watching who had put off having a breast lump looked at, it might spur them on to have it checked out and treated rather than having to go through all the procedures the red-haired woman had been through. Quite unexpectedly, however, I found that I had much more feeling in my new boobs than even the surgeon had said there would be at that stage, and I needed a local anaesthetic to stop me from jumping at the stinging sensation of the buzzing tattoo needles.

The tattoo was extremely bold and dark in colour, but after three weeks the tattoo ink had faded to its true colour.

Yes, I've got to admit it – these breasts are spectacular! They're soft; they wobble, bounce and shimmy. They feel totally natural. It's got nothing to do with suddenly being 'more feminine' – the result is just so mind blowing!

I adore showing off my new boobs – with dignity of course. I've got a habit of extending invitations to interested women to 'have a feel' and I often wear a semi see-through blouse to display my tatts. (I said *tatts!*) Not for the hussy factor, but for the incredible skill, operations and technologies that my body has been able to benefit from, and which is available to all women.

I was asked whether I'd mind talking to a couple of breast cancer ladies about my breast reconstruction experience at a hospital.

Of course out came my tummy cut, and my lovely nippley bosoms for a bit of a shoogle so that the ladies might have a first-hand look at the merchandise they were considering popping into their shopping trolley. They seemed amazed at just how exquisite these babies looked. One lady thought she'd go ahead with it. The other lady winced at the tummy scar and decided the pain wasn't worth it.

I arranged with another breast cancer lady, who was considering reconstruction, to check 'em out. She came to my house and presented me with a box of

Gaye

chocolates, saying, 'I feel like this is asking you to perform some kind of foreplay. I don't have a bunch of flowers, but at least I can give you some chocolates.'

Sandy

A girlfriend in her late 40s had a breast reconstruction and had the colour of the areola tattooed on! Whether it was performed by laser, I don't know. I couldn't imagine her going down to the local tattoo parlour holding her breasts out and saying, 'Here y'are babe, do us a couple of hearts on here!'

I haven't actually seen them, but my friend Pam has.

Pam says, 'You'd never ever know, except that she looks better than any woman our age!'

Diane

Dr Richard had encouraged me to think about having the breast reconstruction from the start. He said, 'It's available. Why don't you go and find out about it?'

I was very much against the idea initially, and when I went in for the mastectomy further surgery was the last thing on my mind. I was adamant. If it wasn't my real breast – my own breast – I wasn't interested.

But because the prosthesis wasn't quite the answer I'd hoped it would be (for me), I did begin to give reconstruction a little bit of thought. I had encouragement from my husband as well; he thought I should do it – or at least go and find out about it.

Both Dr Richard and Alan thought reconstruction would be a good thing. Not that they felt I had to have it or should do it, but they had both been reading me pretty well, and they could see that a prosthesis was a problem for me.

I was very hesitant about doing it because I worried that I might be dissatisfied with the result. But in the end I decided that if it was somewhat 'breast-like' and fitted into my bra without escaping, it was going to be good enough for me. And after all that, if I really didn't like it, I'd simply have it removed.

I did a lot of asking around and finally decided on two plastic reconstructive surgeons, for whom I got referrals.

I originally felt uncomfortable about going to see a plastic surgeon, because I knew it was dealing with a lot of issues for me. One was the fact that I had to go there, undress, and be examined by yet another doctor – and with only one breast, that's not easy. But also I had this belief that a plastic surgeon only deals with the more attractive (the more glamorous) section of the population who are trying to improve their looks, rather than what the surgeon really does which is to help people who have problems with their bodies. In reality, they do all the hard work; they very rarely deal with the beautiful.

But that's how I perceived it, and I thought, 'I'm going in there very fat – one boob and a flesh apron around my stomach.' I really thought that was pushing the boundaries of what this doctor would want to see and do.

I made an appointment with Dr Robert first, and after meeting him knew that he was the person for me. He was unbelievably empathetic, non-judgmental and considerate. I didn't even bother making a comparison appointment with the other referral I had because I felt so confident and comfortable with him.

It was to be at least a two-step operation. The first one was to construct a new breast using tissue from my tummy. Roughly six months later (after the new breast had settled into its proper shape) the surgeon would 'lift' my remaining breast so that it would be in the same position as the new breast. Then, if I wanted it, a nipple would be added during a further small procedure.

I came out of the first operation and was absolutely thrilled with how it looked. It felt and looked wonderful – better than I ever imagined it could. Sure it was uncomfortable in the post-operative days; there's no doubt about that. I did have a few minor complications, but if you asked me whether I would do it all over again, the answer would be, 'Yes, Yes, Yes!'

I don't think it's right for all women – not for a minute. But for those who want to do it, I'd say, 'Go ahead and have it done, because the very worst you could end up with is having to take it off again if you don't like it.'

All up, it's the best thing I've ever done for myself – and I'm talking strictly on a personal basis. I got so much out of the whole business. It wasn't simply a physical change to my body; the transformational change of my attitude was just as phenomenal. I was on the biggest high (other than having my babies) that I've ever had – and it lasted a long, long time. I felt it changed things for me entirely; it changed how I felt about myself.

Both physically and emotionally it was just the biggest thing that has happened to me, ever.

I went back for the second operation six months later. Dr Robert 'lifted' my left breast and made a couple of small adjustments to the reconstructed breast to further improve the shape a little in order to create a 'matched pair'.

Sometime later I returned and had the nipple done. The surgeon took a skin graft from my inside thigh and created it into a nipple and areola for my breast. Having the graft for the nipple means that there's no need for tattooing, due to the 'natural' colour of the graft.

I nearly died when I first saw it though, because – like all things with plastic surgery and reconstructive surgery – it looks different, initially, to how it will look in the end.

At first all I could see was this extremely dark brown nipple. I've got very fair, rather petite nipples and this thing was enormous – very prominent! It would have suited an African tribal woman really well. And I thought, 'I've ruined it; I've blown it big time!'

However, Dr Robert seemed pleased with the result. I didn't say anything to him because I knew he would be mortified to think that I wasn't happy with something he'd done. After he left, one of the nurses noticed my disappointment and said to me, 'It won't stay like that you know; it'll shrink and fade.'

When I got home and had another look I wondered mournfully, 'But just how small can it get, and how pink can it go?' It was so dark. I thought it would never get to the right colour and size to match my other breast, but it has!

So I've got the whole kit and caboodle. And it looks fantastic! So much so, that when I went for a mammogram two years after the reconstruction, the woman who began placing my right breast into the machine interrupted me mid-sentence and contradicted, 'When you're referring to that breast, dear, you don't actually call that a mastectomy – what you've had.'

I paused, slightly confused, and said slowly, 'Yes … I've had a mastectomy.'

'No, no,' she insisted, 'I'll just explain the difference to you. Now, a *mastectomy* is when they take the *whole* breast and a lumpectomy or wedge is when they take only a *part* of your breast. Where you've got those two scars under your breast, that's where your *wedge* has been taken from.'

(This was so insulting, to say the least – like I was a complete and utter idiot and didn't know what surgery I'd had! But in other ways, it was extremely complimentary.)

I said, 'No – that's where my *breast reconstruction* has been placed. I had my tummy taken to replace the whole breast that was removed.'

She was floored. She took this giant gasp of breath and squawked, 'Who did that?'

I told her, 'Dr Robert.'

She was briefly lost for words until she realised how patronising and condescending she had sounded. 'Ohh, I'm so sorry,' she apologised repeatedly, 'but I just can't believe it! I have *never* seen anything better.'

So in the end, I thought it turned out to be an extraordinary compliment. Another uplifting experience.

Doris

The first time I had a breast off, nobody suggested I might care to have half my bottom transplanted onto my chest. I don't think it was even considered in those days. But when the second breast went, my surgeon asked if I wanted to have a think about reconstruction.

There wasn't any point, you know. I mean, I'm perfectly happy to be like this at my age.

Although, with my deep voice, I do get the occasional funny look. When Richard and I are walking along the street, just occasionally someone will hear my voice, look at my flat chest and stare at me as if to say, 'That's a fellow.' Then they'll listen to what I'm actually talking about and realise I am a woman. I get some very daft looks – I must be the fattest transsexual around.

Titbit

To obtain the best results for your bosoms and secure peace of mind, ensure that your reconstructive plastic surgeon is a member of the Australian Society of Plastic Surgeons. (Consult the Society's advertised list of Accredited Surgeons under *Medical Practitioners* in the Telephone Directory.)

CHAPTER 12

The breast time of my life

(Reflections)

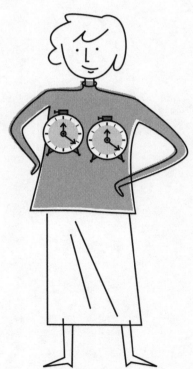

Gaye

I never saw my sense of humour during cancer as some sort of laugh therapy – but the absolute joy of spirit I owned and embraced was extremely thera-peutic. And I think it also helped those connected with me to learn about something horrible in a way they weren't used to. Not that helping everyone else cope was my initial aim – but it did seem to help defuse a lot of the agony and help people re-evaluate the conventional stigma surrounding breast cancer.

Reliable, factual information was a wonderful asset during this time. I tried to make sure that any problems were addressed; I asked to see medical reports relating to my case and was given copies. With each new doctor or specialist we told them that we wanted everything to be explained simply and clearly. They did. I did as much homework as I needed to so that my choices were made with clear understanding of each situation. I didn't want any regrets. When it was all over and done I didn't want to say, 'I should have done this' or 'I should have done that ...'

I didn't plan on having cancer — I just planned to make the most out of it. I never considered my breast cancer to be a crisis or an ordeal.

A friend recently explained the Chinese meaning of 'crisis' to me as 'a time of changing'. 'A changing in the cycle of life, a changing in the cycle of time. It holds possibilities – of a good danger or bad danger; life or death. Nobody knows what it will be. You have the opportunity to take it and change it to something good – something valuable.'

To me this is so profound. There are possibilities in every circumstance. Each circumstance provides the opportunity and potential for good or bad, and we make our choice, allowing one way or the other to prosper.

So maybe my breast cancer was a 'crisis' after all – because while I could see the aspects of potential danger and possible death, it was also possible to transform the available opportunities into something wonderful – into a celebration of living.

I remain grateful for the experience.

It's ironic, but the 'time out' it provided helped me to discover so much about myself that I certainly would not have learnt had I not gone through it. It has enriched my life immeasurably and I have been given back so much more than what was taken from me. My physical changes are nothing compared with the mental changes. I faced a fear that I'd carried since childhood – that cancer was death. I was cast into the eye of a swirling hurricane, but it turned out I was just whizzing round on the washing line having the time of my life. (Frowned upon by some; but it's just so much fun!)

I had happiness, but I had much more. I had true joy.

I held it. I embraced it. I owned it – deep in my heart and my being.

Cancer affirmed life and became the celebration of being.

Sandy

Having cancer has been one of the most wonderful experiences of my life, simply because of all the lovely things that have happened to me along the way. From that little bit of bad I've had a wealth of joy and happiness – thanks to my husband and my children.

I've been fortunate to meet so many wonderful people, talk with them, and share something that is very, very special.

It's difficult to convey this to someone who hasn't had the disease (with all its experiences) because they really just don't understand. They say they understand it, and I'm sure they try to understand it as far as they can, but they can never relate to the intimacy that people who have the disease can share.

Some things just happen to you, I believe, for a reason. I think you're put to a test and you have choices. And you've got to make it an absolute winner!

Diane

My self-esteem was rock bottom before I had my cancer and mastectomy – which certainly brought me down that bit further. But from all of that, I've gained much more than I've lost. I've gained so much from the emotional things and the people I've met. I've gained *enormously*! I've got a new and better self – and self-esteem – than I ever had before.

At times I see people devastated over something small. I can sit back and be sympathetic and empathetic with them, but inside I'm thinking, 'You have got to be joking! That is so pathetically trivial. Why would you be in a complete and utter state over something that is so immaterial to life?!' (Like 'Ohh no-o-o, the car's got a scratch!' 'I can't get that dress in *blue*! I don't want the other colours; I want *blue*!')

Really? It's that big a deal?!

To me, the trivial became more trivial and the important became more important.

My expressions of thanks could never truly convey my gratitude to my husband, family, friends doctors and nurses – in fact, all the people I had contact with over this time. They all helped me in more ways than they could ever imagine, and I feel so fortunate to have experienced such wonderful support and love. I feel

Diane

very strongly that the surgery and medical treatment I had was beneficial in my recovery but it was the support, love and care that made the difference.

To have wonderful doctors was such a great gift. Dr Bill, Dr Richard, Dr Jacquie and Dr Robert made an enormous difference to my overall outcome. They took care of the 'whole' me – not just the physical me. I love them all.

Doris

I think it's useful to have a 'near miss' in life, because cancer has made me see a lot of things differently. It made me more appreciative.

I've always been fat you see, and I've always hated being fat – and when Richard, my wonderful second husband, made it clear that our relationship was more than just friendship, I wondered, 'How will he cope? I'm ten years older than he is, I have two children, I'm fat, and I only have one breast. I can cope with it, but can he?'

He coped with it beautifully, and it made me feel very loving about Richard (that a man can be so gentle and so accepting) because I don't know whether I

Doris

could ever be that accepting about things. It was an special extra reason to fall in love with Richard – and I did.

Another thing it showed me was that I am less scared of death than I was before I had cancer. It made me think about it a lot; I still do of course. I'm getting to the age where I should! But here I am teaching – in a new career at 74! And at least I know I'll never die of breast cancer!

180   *Bosom Buddies*

Thanks
for the mammaries

I feel truly privileged to have met so many wonderful people. I have felt the love and support of family and friends, and seen beauty inside the hearts of strangers.

I would like to acknowledge and extend my thanks to everyone who took part in the experience.

Thank you.

Foremost to my Father God for allowing me the honour of this experience – Thank you for giving me the wings to soar high.

Thank you my darling Stephen, Elissa and Kerrie for teaching me to use those wings to fly.

Thanks, love and kisses to my Mum, Dad and sisters – and all my wonderful family, relatives and breast friends for prayers, cards, flowers, help and messages of love. Your support uplifted me like the proverbial underwire bra.

Thank you, Jim and Sandy, Alan and Diane, Richard and Doris and families, for allowing us inside your experiences, emotions, courage and resolve.

You are remarkable people.

Many thanks to everyone who helped to make this book a reality. Thanks to Melbourne comedians Christine Basil; Linda Haggar and Fayer Younger for help in compiling the 'Top 10 Reasons' list.

Breast wishes
Gaye

Resources

The Cancer Council Australia
National Information Line
Phone 13 11 20
(This number is the cost of a local call and transfers you directly to
the Cancer Council in your state.)
GPO Box 4708, Sydney NSW 2001
Level 4, 70 William Street, East Sydney NSW 2011
Phone 9380 9022
Fax 9380 9033
Email info@cancer.org.au
Website www.cancer.org.au

BreastScreen Australia
A joint Commonwealth/State and Territory program, BreastScreen
Australia offers free mammograms to women over 50.
Phone 13 20 50
Email phd.frontdesk@health.gov.au
Website www.breastscreen.info.au

Bosom Buddies Inc.
An ACT organisation that provides support for women with breast
cancer.
Phone 0419 698 188
Email www.bosombuddies.com.au

Breast Cancer Support Network
This organisation is a network of consumer groups and individuals
which links Australians who have been personally affected by breast
cancer.
Ms Lyn Swinburne – National Coordinator
P.O. Box 4082
AUBURN SOUTH VIC. 3122
Phone (03) 9805 2500
Fax (03) 9805 2599
Email beacon@bcna.org.au

The Young Ones
This group offers support to women under 45 years who have
experienced breast cancer. The group is a member of Breast Cancer
Network Australia and is based in Collingwood, Victoria.
Phone (03) 9330 2785 or 0411 235 964
Email tanya_wilson@optusnet.com.au
Website www.ezia.net.au/theyoungones